E.L. STEPHENSON
3348 N. Thompson • Site 38
Springdale, AR 72764
(501) 750-1236

Over the Hill at 60
and

Picking Up Speed!

E.L. Stephenson

E.L. STEPHENSON

Over the Hill at 60
and
Picking Up Speed!

My Office Publishing Company
1417 Eton St.
Fayetteville, Arkansas 72703

ISBN: 0-9654107-0-6

Editing, Typography, and Design:
Jan Cooper · My Office Publishing Co.
(501) 575-0135

PRINTED IN THE UNITED STATES OF AMERICA

DEDICATION

This book is dedicated to the two million people each year who believe society's lies about our being over the hill at 60 and there is not much left in life after 65 but to wait for the undertaker who will put them under the hill before they reach 75.

It is dedicated to all of those who are looking for a road map that will lead them to the joys of exploring the harvest years of their lives after retirement and who believe that every birthday signals another year in which they can have more fun than in the last.

It is first and foremost, however, dedicated to George Burns who refused to go over the hill or under it, let alone both. He went around the hill and made fun for himself and for the world for 100 years, then spent 7 weeks deciding whether to rejoin Gracie or to go for 120 years or 970. Gracie won. All of us can follow his example.

E. J. Stephenson

3348 N. Thompson, Site 38
Springdale, AR 72764
(501) 750-1236

The wonderful world of retirement is what you choose to make it. It is mostly a do-it-yourself job, and as with most other tasks we undertake in our lives, there are a myriad of paths we can take to reach our goals. Positive thinkers always look until they find the bright side. Sure, their friends and family members have died off or, in many cases, moved away, but the positive thinkers see that their enemies are also gone. They find the bright side, then they set about to find new friends and avoid making new enemies.

Contrary to society's myths, retirement is not where you go to wait for the undertaker to put you under the hill soon after everyone tells you you're over it. Retirement is payday for the graduates of life's boot camp where you learned <u>how</u> to have a full life and have fun. It is your reward for raising your family, working hard, and planning for the future.

Abe Lincoln hit the nail on the head when he said, "Most people are about as happy as they make up their minds to be." Abe knew that our mental attitude controls our happiness and our misery. Never in our lives is that so true as in our retirement years. But if we were all as smart as we know how to be, we would all be perfect and every day would be perfectly and gloriously happy. It could be done, but do we want it? Not really. A few fleas are good for a dog. They keep him from getting lazy and bored. If every day of our lives was perfectly happy, we would soon tire of the monotony. The sour grapes make the sweet ones taste better. The storms make the sunshine seem brighter.

At 96 — after two careers, over a million and a half miles in 49 automobiles, over 4,000 hours flying airplanes, a few thousand miles running rivers in boats, duck/goose/pheasant hunting, shooting high-powered rifles, and a thousand other ways of having fun — my life began at 90 when I started exploring how to stay young. I found 45,000 books and articles on how to grow old that our horse-and-buggy society uses to train[1] us to be over the hill and 60 and under it at 74. Thirty-one percent of all of us who reach 60 choose that route and ask no questions. We mavericks in the 69% who ignore the life expectancy we are told is our destiny ask why.

The "Stay Young Land" is where we can spend the half century or more past 70. It is a place where we can use the knowledge and experience we spent 70 years acquiring. All of us who have survived past 75 are proud of the accomplishment, but I believe I am the first one to recognize it for what it is and what we can do with it. Most of us wander in this Stay Young Land beyond 75 like lost Gypsies in an overnight camp. We do not know what to make of it, so we wander aimlessly through life wondering why we're still here, why the undertaker hasn't shown up to take us away.

Never in history has anyone explored a more fantastic and fascinating place than the Stay Young Land, and I am delighted to share with you what I have discovered and why I am committed to staying just as long as I can.

Thinking that we can outlive our life expectancy can put us in command of our own lives and destinies. We know that our lives are what we make them, happy or miserable, productive or stagnant, giving or taking, accepting or questioning. We know that we have to continue living and growing and working at making this world a little better place for everyone or there will be no point in staying here.

I have discovered that positive thinking people who recognize and accept that society has placed upon them the idea of "being old and useless" can cut through the negative impact society's teachings have had and choose for themselves to stay here as long as they want to.

The most important thing I've learned in my quest is that a positive mental attitude portrayed by all of us who have chosen to send the undertaker from our doors can and will cure the negative thinking of society, given time.

As humans, we should aim for perfection and aim high and be happy nearly all the time. As long as we are humans, we can never become quite perfect. There will always be some unfinished business. Goals for humans cannot be fixed, nor should they be. They should always be raised. That makes us continue to grow. When we quit growing, we start dying.

Nothing is ever done unless you think it can be done. If you think it is impossible, it is. It is up to us to prove the power of mental attitude by letting the tortoise — medical science — plod along while we put our money on the hare — mental attitude — and raise life expectancy to 100 in one generation. Okay. It may turn out to be expecting too much too soon, but it costs nothing to try, and we will have more fun than if we hadn't tried.

— E.L. Stephenson
1996 (96 years young)

———

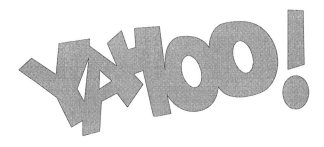

The *Wall Street Journal* of October 16, 1992, told us that in 1950, a 65-year-old man had a 7% chance of reaching 90. Today, he has a 25% chance. That means 1 out of 14 then, 1 out of 4 now.

The article went on to say that entomologists at the University of California who hatch millions of Mediterranean fruit flies to release to protect fruit crops have been surprised at how they die. Their death rate is highest at 40 days of life. Fifteen percent die at day 40, then it levels off and then decreases. Those who reach 100 days or older have a daily risk of dying of 4 to 6 percent. That is less than the death rate for 20-day-old flies. Now there's a push-up for your brain. It is also a picker-upper for your mental attitude.

Obviously, there are positive thinkers and negative thinkers among Mediterranean flies, just as among us humans, and mental attitude also controls their life span. I began to wonder if their percentages are about the same as ours, and I learned that 31% of those who are healthy at 60 die within 15 years. Only 69% survive past 75 to enjoy life's harvest time. They are the positive thinkers.

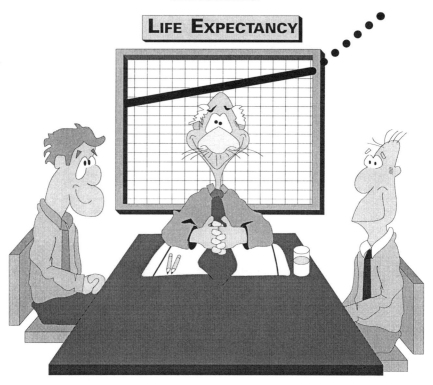

Negative thinkers often say they do not want to live after their friends and families are gone. Positive thinkers always look on the bright side. We know there are others we can love and enjoy during the years we choose to keep living.

Those of us who choose to dare to use the brains our Creator has given us and make our own decisions and open the doors of opportunity to a freer and fuller life begin realizing that life is what we make it and that we are expected to do something worthwhile with it.

***We are beginning to see that
life begins at retirement.***

It is a reincarnation, a second chance, an opportunity to do all the things we've dreamed of doing but did not have the time.

Ask yourself this question: Why is it that in every other of life's endeavors, reaching the Senior level is to reach the pinnacle, the sought after grail, but when someone becomes a Senior Citizen and retires, they are suddenly viewed as non-thinking, non-functioning, non-contributing human beings? You will immediately begin to see that society's perception of "being old" has nothing to do with ability — it only has to do with a number on a calendar.

Spreading life over more years means we can have more fun as we go along. We can experiment more and try new things, even new careers. We have begun seeing that loads of things can be accomplished in the extra half century we are choosing to live.

We no longer think of retirement as a sudden change from work to play. We have quit wondering when we're going to die and are planning how to pack as many years as possible with a full life. We have discovered that there are no spectators in retirement, so we stay busy at anything useful and maintain the interest in life without which we would die. We have learned that golf and fishing are not a full life, so we are following Danny Thomas' advice more and more and volunteering to help others not so fortunate. We are heeding the words of George Burns who told us that "growing old" might be inevitable but that we do not have to "become old."

We believe we were created as thinking, productive human beings, not robots or slaves, so we work at remaining independent and contributing members of society. We believe our Creator expected us to make our own decisions, learn and grow and be all that we can be and leave the world a little better than we found it. We believe He wanted us to be happy and productive helpers, not disgruntled, complaining parasites.

We are delighted to learn that while the rate of deaths per year per thousand keeps rising rapidly to 74, it quits rising there and decreases rapidly. We know that means that a 110 year old is no more likely to die this year than an 74 year old. We have noticed that the hills are getting steeper each year, but we decide to take a new lease on life. We know that if we can take what life hands out at 74, we can probably go right on to 120. Consider this:

At 74, 79% survive at least one year.

At 84, 83% survive at least one year.

At 94, 93% survive at least one year.

At 104, 99.47% survive at least one year.

At 114, 99.95% survive at least one year.

HALLELUJAH! HALLELUJAH!

These figures were compiled at my request by The Bankers Life and Casualty Company, Merchandise Mart Plaza, in Chicago. They have carried my supplemental Medicare coverage for many years — at a lower price and with a more business-like, on-their-toes attitude than three previous carriers I have had. All the census figures I could find lumped everyone over 85 into one group, apparently expecting everyone to die then . . . if not sooner.

I THINK; THEREFORE, I CAN!

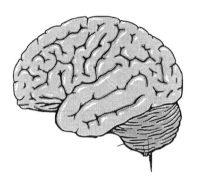

The human brain is the most magnificent and wonderful miracle on the face of our Earth. It can grab a handful of stars with positive thinking, or it can become bogged down in a dismal swamp of despair with negative thinking. It controls our happiness and our misery — and sets the date for far too many funerals too soon. The tremendous power of positive thinking can be harnessed to control everything in our everyday lives. It can control maybe half of our health and almost all of our ability to enjoy life.

It is interesting that man has always had a brain and has always lived in a world full of goodies that went relatively unrecognized for most of his history. Except for some moon dust and rocks, everything that is on this Earth now has always been here for us to discover and use to our benefit, but it has only been recently that man's eyesight has improved to the point that he has "discovered" them and converted them into the marvelous tools and products that make our lives so rich today.

We humans were very slow to see the opportunities available — and even slower at times to see the broader possibilities of what was right in front of our noses. For example, a thousand years before Christ, the Chinese invented "toys" called rockets. Nearly 30 centuries later, we rode them to the moon — after Hitler showed us how. The opportunities for mankind that the "toy" had always held were finally, after 3000 years, recognized and harnessed.

In the first century, Hero invented a steam engine in Alexandria. Hero's steam engine was also seen as a fascinating toy. In 1829, George Stephenson used one to outrun a horse for the first time. In 1941, Whittle recognized that Hero's engine was jet propelled and put one on a plane. It only took half a century then for jet propelled planes to travel from L.A. to Washington, D.C. in 68 minutes, 1120 years after jet propulsion was invented. Today, some planes fly at Mach III, three times the speed of sound, and we have ridden rockets to the moon at 24,000 miles per hour, a speed that will soon be increased by nuclear rockets.

These remarkable results have been accomplished in just over a century, but the raw materials and technology were available to all the men who came before us for centuries.

Unlike the cow that jumped over the moon, our generation finally landed and walked on it.

It had taken mankind ever since Adam to get into the air, then it took only half a century to travel into space. In a century and a half, we have gone from the speed of a horse to over 24,000 miles an hour. We have put the atom to work, and we expect nuclear rockets to put men on Mars and to visit other planets in our children's and grandchildren's lifetimes.

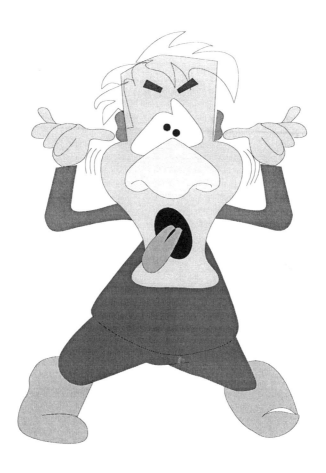

The myths surrounding the
so-called aging process deserve the very
best you have to give them!

You haven't seen much yet, however. We are just getting started. In December of 1996, our space probe Galileo traveled 2.3 million miles in the past six years and is now circling Jupiter for the next two years. It needed to check Jupiter's temperature which scientists believed was 22,000 degrees Fahrenheit. Galileo dropped a 750-pound probe traveling 106,000 miles per hour toward Jupiter 130,000 miles away. It confirmed the 22,000 degrees Fahrenheit before it burned up. Now Galileo can be sure of just how close it can safely get to Jupiter.

Rocket scientists are the best brains
we have developed in 167 years.
Hallelujah! Hallelujah!
Now we can fire Congress and hire
one rocket scientist to do what
Congress doesn't seem to be able to do.

Can you blame me for wanting to stick around to see the next 20-some-odd years? In my early years, we used kerosene lamps, though Wabash, Indiana, and New York City had installed the first electric lights in 1885. We had wash-boards and galvanized steel wash tubs and a few hand-cranked washers. We often made our own soap. There was nationwide telegraph and some local phone service in some towns, but I remember reading of the first transcontinental phone call when I was in the eighth grade. Men's dress shirts had celluloid collars. They had to go to a steam laundry to be cleaned for three cents each. They were the first plastic items.

Some of the newer cooking utensils were alumi-num. The first aluminum ever made is the tiny pyramid on the top of the Washington Monument. The first auto visited our town in 1903. The first Nickelodeon black-and-white movie came about the same time. Wireless was 12 years old when it brought news of the Titanic sinking in 1912. Radio came in 1920. Every town had a livery stable where you could rent horse-drawn buggies and carriages. About 1910, new buggies had rounded corners on the two seat corners and were called "auto-type seats." There were a few single-cylinder gasoline or kerosene engines with big flywheels with pulleys and belts. One engine could power all the machines in a small shop. Corn shellers and sorghum mills to press juice out of cane stalks were powered by one or more horses walking around in circles pulling a wooden beam like one spoke in a wheel. Compare that to the wonders we are witness to today, and you'll see that watching the years go by is fun if you stay young. It is also the "Greatest Show on Earth," as P.T. Barnum called his circus.

Until 1829, we humans either walked at about three miles per hour, rode horses or mules, or rode in carts and wagons drawn by some animal. Cave men, the Romans, and even America's colonists had shelter, food, and clothing of only slightly improving quality though thousands of years separated them. Man had learned to build a fire, make a wheel, plant crops, and read and write — we knew little else until 1829, when George Stephenson put his steam locomotive on a track and discovered — again — one of the first notable inventions that propelled humankind into looking for more ways to improve our existence.

Stephenson called his locomotive "The Rocket" after the Chinese toy. Suddenly humans traveled faster than ever before. At last, man began to comprehend that God gave him legs but did not teach him to walk, that He gave man eyes but did not teach him to see, that He gave us brains but did not teach us to think. Always He left the discovering of His gifts up to us, and we only began to really open our eyes after we grasped the true potential of jet engines and rockets — some two or three thousand years after they were invented.

Outrunning a horse in Stephenson's locomotive had a miraculous effect on us, and we began wondering — and looking — for other possibilities Mother Earth had to offer to make our tomorrows better. This event sounded reveille for civilization and became a most significant milestone in the growth of man. At that juncture, our civilization really began, and the Great Easter Egg Hunt for more surprises that was launched in 1829 is still picking up speed.

Here is a partial list of goodies found in just the last 169 years:

Reaper	1831
Pneumatic tire	1845
Sewing machine	1846
Typewriter	1867
Internal combustion engine	1867
Dynamite	1867
Barbed wire	1873
Electric motor	1873
Telephone	1876
Phonograph	1877
Incandescent light	1879
Gasoline-powered automobile	1885
Diesels	1892
Zippers	1893
Radio	1895
X-Ray	1895
Wireless	1900
Air conditioning	1902

Airplane	1903
Helicopter	1907
Television	1920
Rocket potential	1947
Nuclear reaction	1942
Four-minute mile	1954
Space travel	1957
Lasers	1960
Moon landing	1969

(Pressure cooker — 1645, believe it or not!)

Some of the inventions were grabbed immediately and put to work, like barbed wire, but some took many years to be accepted and used. Remember, the benefits of the steam engine took 1700 years and rockets took 3000 years for man to catch onto to after they were invented.

Not content, however, with our mind's present ability to think, some smart scientists think the mind's ability to control the body to which it is attached can be increased. One university has ordered 200 machines to be used by athletes to help their minds order muscles to perform better. One high jumper used one for two months while training and jumped five inches higher than ever before. The scientists are satisfied that it works. Now they are looking for side effects.

The Twentieth Century brought the airplane in 1903; it and rapid communication brought global competition. Now everyone in the world has to compete with every other person.

Competition — good or bad — brings about progress. The tougher, the better. Without it, you have a post office.

In 1954, another major event occurred when Roger Bannister ran the first 4-minute mile any human had ever run. Roger was evidently the first to really <u>think</u> he could — so he did. Down through the ages, probably thousands had tried and failed, but within two years of Roger's making the 4-minute mile, 317 others did it. Today, over 800 have done it.

> *Roger proved to us that*
> *if you <u>think</u> you can do a thing,*
> *think it to your core, <u>you can</u>.*

Of course, you may say he just had an extraordinarily positive mental attitude. You bet he did. Mental attitude controls almost every aspect of our lives, and each of us as an individual chooses if that attitude is positive or negative. Many of the people who think and act negatively know it, but nobody does anything about it. Mental attitude is a little like the weather, except it can be controlled or changed.

Like everything else, the more you know about mental attitude, the better it works. I got my first lesson when I enlisted in the Marine Corps in World War I and was sent to boot camp on Parris Island, South Carolina. The drill instructors were perfectionists, who tried hard to hammer into our heads that we could do anything we thought we could do — provided we thought we could and were willing to do whatever was necessary to learn how. Signs reading "If you don't know, you get killed" were posted everywhere. After it was over, I was grateful. It helped prepare me for the boot camp of life, from which I was graduated at about 70 years of age.

The one thing that Marine boot camp didn't tell me,

however, is that society was lying to me about being over the hill at 60.

You do not have to be a scientist to explore "impossible" things. No wonder we have doubled the amount of knowledge in the world in the last 25 years. Now that the information highway is knocking at our door, it will double again in less than 25 years. All of this will be the reward for all of us who choose to use our brains, and this is only the beginning. Our Creator is not the only one who is happy.

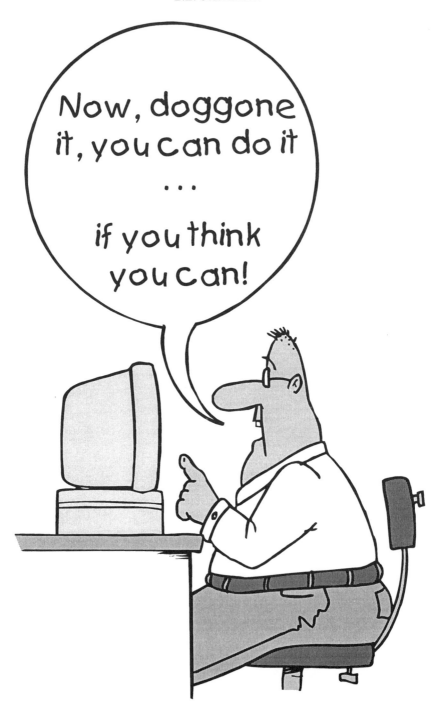

Silly and Stupid?

Learned scholars impress upon us that we humans have never explored, let alone used, 95% of our brain's capacity. To prove how silly and stupid we are, they cite examples like this:

> *For at least 3,000 years, rats have tormented humans and are still doing so. Man has not found a remedy. We have known for a long time that there are no rats where there are no people. Are we too stupid to stop feeding them?*

We send Seniors to Florida in their later years to show them we love them and are trying to be as nice to them as we, in our turn, hope to be treated. When they get there, they learn that Florida is called "God's Waiting Room." That label was no doubt pinned on it by its Chamber of Commerce who mistakenly thought that it would attract tourists. Or perhaps some bureaucrat in the vast "aging process" thought what a beautiful slogan it would be for the assisted suicide of Seniors. Dr. Kevorkian does not assist healthy people to end their lives. Society's method is only a little better than Hitler's, but the results are the same.

Seniors are told, albeit through deed rather than words, that they are at death's door and that it may be opened any minute for them to be pulled in. Constantly reminding a person that he is about to die is hardly the best way to keep him alive. Many a rich uncle has been sent to God's Waiting Room by a loving nephew who was having difficulty waiting for his inheritance.

We talk a lot about living full and happy lives and getting the most out of it. Then most of us work every day for the undertakers. We do it for no pay, without being asked and without being needed. Undertakers are remarkable people and great salesmen. They are the only sales people in the world who can sit on their fannies and wait for prospects to come to them. They are the only sales people in the world who make money off prospects before the sale is closed. Other salesmen say, "Buy now, pay later." Undertakers say, "Pay now, die later." They call it by its high-tech name: Pre-arrangement. Undertakers have no collection problems and no trouble satisfying customers who never complain and never talk back.

I am not poking fun just at undertakers. I am poking fun at our whole society and its ideas about the aging process. But now that you have seen that even undertakers have a funny side, it can start you down a path of looking for the bright side in everything. Having gently roasted the undertakers, though, I will now point out how they earn their keep and our everlasting gratitude.

Undertakers can put a peaceful expression or even a victory smile on the faces of our loved ones who died in pain. They give us a memory that we can keep forever while our memory of our loved one's last hours mercifully fade away. We are grateful.

That doesn't mean, however, that we are obligated to expedite our own funerals in order to make the undertakers feel needed and add to their pocketbooks.

We really do expedite our own and one another's funerals in hundreds of ways by negative remarks like, "How are you feeling, Bill?" It would have cost no more to have said, "Gee, Bill, you look great today." It is not necessary to stick to absolute truth. The road to happiness is paved in many places with little white lies. You would not tell your bride that her cooking is terrible, that her taste in clothes is pitiful. You would not tell your friend that his choice of cars is poor, that he's not bright enough for a job he wants. All of us could brighten our world give everyone, including ourselves, a lift. When you tell Joe, "Better slow down. You're not as young as you used to be," you mean well, but you are expediting his funeral and yours. No one thinks they are in any way expediting their own funeral, but consider for a moment remarks like, "Well, I'm about as good as I can be for my age."

See how it works? Start looking for things to compliment in everything — attitude, manners, clothing, grooming, capacity for work — anything and everything that is better than the ordinary should be complimented. Make it a point to lift the spirits of everyone you meet, and you can't help but lift your own in the process. And the miracle is that once we lift someone else's spirits, they are much more apt to turn around and pass that good feeling on to the next person they encounter. Smile, get to work, and make your own sunshine, but go one step further and share it with all you meet.

Always keep your eyes on the future — yours and everyone with whom you communicate. You can't do anything about the past. Your present-day bed is made, but your future bed could probably use a new bedspread and some new, fluffy pillows. You will be utterly amazed how contagious positive thinking/acting/talking/living can be. Even if someone gives you a one-finger salute, thank him for pointing out that you're number one.

After you pass 74 and realize that the hills no longer get steeper every year, each birthday becomes happier and more and more fun, your enthusiasm begins to bubble over. It begins to rub off on those who have considered you a brain-dead non-person who should have been buried long ago. Some of them try, and a few succeed, to realize that they have been wrong and begin treating you like a person again. If they manage to reach this level, they usually begin to envy you. That's good. It makes them start thinking about reaching for higher goals for themselves.

Continually reminding anyone that the end is near is the fastest way to make it so. If we spent as much time planning a happy future as we do contemplating death, we would all survive to 120 or more. Silly and stupid? Perhaps the learned scholars know more about us than we can accept about ourselves.

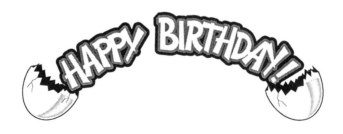

POSITIVE THINKING
IS A
SALES PITCH!

I've always been a salesman. The better I showed others how to make their tomorrows better, the better I ate. Almost everything I've learned in my life about selling, I learned the first day I tried, and since that day, I have learned only one other thing of importance — to correct other people's mistakes. With those two gems of wisdom, I made a good living for myself.

I believe I was eight and a skinny kid who could eat one-third of his weight in food while running all day. An older brother and I went out in the lumber wagon about 1908 with a small load of two or three hundred heads of cabbage. We were headed for Fredonia, Kansas, a town of nearly 4,000 then as now, to sell them house to house. In those days, cabbage had a shelf life in a store of two days or maybe three, then it was no longer saleable.

We drove streets all over town. I rang the doorbells on one side of the street with a head of cabbage in my hand. Later, I would carry one of two pounds and a bigger one, maybe as big as ten or more pounds. My brother worked the other side of the street, all dirt or gravel but no paving. The team needed no driver. They kept up with us

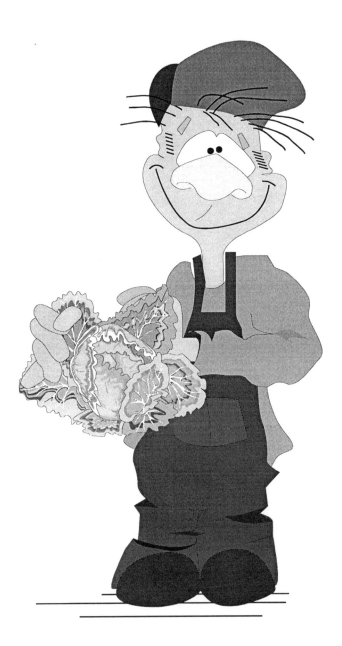

as we went from house to house. There were only three or four automobiles in town.

When a housewife came to her door, I would show her a small head of cabbage for a nickel and a bigger one, if I had two, for a dime. I would tell her it had been cut after sundown the day before and was really fresh. Our percentage of sales to calls I would guess to be well over 50%. I knew nothing about selling. All I did was give the housewives the honest facts and let them see the cabbage and sell themselves. I did not know then that the best way to sell anything is to give the customer all the facts and make it as easy as possible for him or her to come to a decision. In other words, help people only a little to sell themselves, then they will stay. When they buy, you know they will always be your customer unless you let them down in some way.

Many, many years later, after reading all the books I could find on selling, it dawned on me that I had learned the easiest and best way to sell with those heads of cabbage. The only other bit of wisdom I had to add to that was learning that by correcting my competitors' mistakes on airport insurance policies, I let the owner buy my product. I made no effort to close the sale.

We 69% who choose to live positively and long must all be salesmen now. We will close sales right and left by being positive, by being role models, by sharing what we have learned on our own, as well as what we have chosen not to believe.

Positive and honest salesmanship cannot help but convince at least half of the 31% who haven't discovered the truth to stay with us to enjoy more of those golden years after retirement.

Good salesmen earn their keep and can be proud of what they have done and are doing to build brighter tomorrows. However, all of us know a few salesmen whose sole purpose in life seems to be attempting to sell us things we do not need and that are downright harmful to our quality of life. Salesmen of society's myths fall into this category because it seems that, while everything else is picking up speed today, society's negative, dreary outlook on aging is the same old snake oil routine. The reason is perfectly clear — once you see it.

We seldom harbor a negative thought about the nice people who are involved in the "good" of the community. They run schools, churches, charities, clubs, and practically everything else. We never think of people in the private sector as bureaucrats, but they are. They are well-paid, have perks and pensions, and few are overworked. They fight all change. Change, any change, might upset their apple carts, rock their boats, and endanger their jobs or hobbies. They protect their jobs, as all humans do. Even the dedicated ones, and there are many, protect their jobs.

The bureaucrats who brainwash us with their negative thinking would be better off if they would switch to positive thinking. If they were positive thinkers — and they would probably all tell you they are — they would teach Seniors to look ahead to nice things and the bright side. They could make you as happy as you were as a child waiting for Santa Claus. Instead, they keep trying to smooth the road to graves. Just paving the road to the cemetery makes dying easier, but it wastes enormous effort

that could be better spent by thinking positively and helping Seniors stay young and useful to society.

It only took human beings two or three years to
build an atom bomb. We chartered the American Cancer
Society in 1913 to find a cure for cancer, a charter which is
to expire when a cure is found. Each year, we are told that
success is expected very soon. We throw more money at
it, but not many humans can fire themselves by doing the
job they were hired to do. Another way to state it is to say
that no money can be made by finding a cure for cancer.
Consequently, the same minds with the same technologies
and information available, can produce an instrument of
mass destruction but not find a cure for this horrible disease. Many bureaucrats, like researchers, are hired to do a
job, which, if they do it, ends the job. They learn to be
constantly on guard.

In the past, society has had a lot of help from Seniors themselves in their assisted suicides because Seniors
have been as misinformed and confused as the rest of the
population. Everyone, including Seniors, has conceded
that the world belongs to the young after we tire of it — or
it tires of us.

Society started to teach us to brainwash one another
in hundreds of ways when we were very young. Remember, society told us there was no Santa Claus, and we went
out and told our friends, and they told their friends. As we
grew and watched our elders, we learned that when we
reached retirement age, we were "supposed" to inquire
about one another's aches and pains and to compare them,
all the while working for the undertakers, without pay and
without being asked. You could say we were taught to
pimp for the undertakers.

We were told to work hard and earn a rest at retirement. We were treated, and we treated one another, as humans in possession of all our faculties. The day we retired, however, even from the head of a business, we became non-persons, no longer capable of managing our own affairs on the downhill slide to our graves. We had to "grow old" like everybody inevitably does. People began treating us kindly, in their opinion, and wanted to keep us comfortable while our brains were dying. They thought nothing of making an appointment or promise of some kind and then breaking it without apology. After all, we were no longer people. We got the respect a vegetable might get.

Even people, otherwise intelligent and nearing retirement age themselves, are as guilty as anyone else. Of course, there is a small minority who never feel that stupid. Even part of the already retired are guilty, and so are some doctors. But those of us who decline society's offer of assisted suicide beyond 75 are still on life's stage and intend to stay here, come hell or high water. We whipped society when we dared survive beyond 75, and we can do it again. We are sick and tired of seeing our friends lied to and persuaded to accept a funeral date they can postpone, as we did, and help us explore and map this most glorious time of our lives.

Inspiration from any source is like a swig from the fountain of youth to all ages.

Our history is full of sagas of people who could inspire others to do heroic things. Most of them took place in exciting surroundings like battlefields, fires, calamities, etc. Far fewer involved only one man or a small group.

Miracles are made of ordinary ideas put together in the right order, and everyone is hungry for a ray of hope for the future, and history is full of loners who changed the world. Most are just ordinary people like the Wright Brothers in Dayton, Ohio.

If you are in need of some inspiration, just look at these Seniors who have moved forward with their lives long after society would have had them dead and buried:

- At 99, David Eugene Ray of Franklin, Tennessee, started to learn to read.

- At 99, Mieczyslaw Horsczowski, the classical pianist, recorded a new album.

- At 98, ceramist Beatrice Wood exhibited her latest work.

- At 97, Martin Miller of Indiana was working full-time as a lobbyist for Senior citizens.

- At 96, Kathrine Robinson Everett was practicing law in North Carolina.

- At 94, comedian George Burns performed at Proctor's Theater in Schenectady, New York — 63 years after he first played there.

- At 93, actress Dame Judith Anderson gave a one-hour benefit performance.

- At 92, Paul Spangler completed his fourteenth marathon.

- At 91, Hulda Crooks climbed Mt. Whitney, the highest mountain in the continental United States.

- At 88, Doris Eaton Travis graduated from the University of Oklahoma with a degree in history.

- At 87, Mary Baker Eddy founded the Christian Science Monitor.

- At 87, mystery writer Phyllis Whitney published her seventy-first book, *The Singing Stones*.

- At 84, Ed Benham ran a marathon in 4 hours, 17 minutes, 51 seconds.

- At 84, Amos Alonzo Stagg coached the College of the Pacific football team.

- At 83, baby doctor Benjamin Spock was arrested at Cape Canaveral, Florida, for demonstrating on behalf of world peace.

Look around your own hometown. My guess is you can find many other names to add to this list, Seniors quietly going about their work and lives, living happy and contributing to their communities, far too busy to be thinking about when the undertaker will come for them.

Professor Goddard reached for the stars and made it possible for man to visit them. Now, 12 Americans have walked on the moon, and we are planning a trip to Mars. It took us thousands of years to get into the air and another half century to get into space. Can you think of a more magnificent inspiration? What one man can do, others can do.

Don't worry about not being able to find a job.

After 70, every task is a delight because you DON'T HAVE TO DO IT.

You can thumb your nose at it, or you can let it wait until you are darn well ready to do it. You can pick and choose what you want to do.

We saw Alf Landon, candidate for president in 1936, when the Reagans stopped in Kansas City to congratulate him on his 100th birthday. On TV he looked very alive, and it is a shame that the Reagans did not plant the idea in his head to go to 120. He probably could have made it.

If Alf Landon at 100 and Irving Berlin at 101 had been given a reason to want to go on living, they could be with us yet. Both were very helpful, public-spirited men. If someone had pointed out to them that they were influential role models who could become even more helpful to humanity by hanging on and postponing their own funerals, they might have believed they should live a lot more years. Just showing them that they could still help others and be inspirations might well have given them the all important reason to go on living and giving. Without it, people die regardless of their years.

Postponing your own funeral gets easier with practice, and helping others do the same will help you postpone yours even longer. When you find a retiree who thinks he is nearing the end, raise his sights, urge him to aim higher by setting a new goal of 100, 120, or 970. The price is the same for all three. All it requires is thinking you can. Remember, thinking you can gets easier with practice.

In 1992, Sam Walton, who had fought bone cancer for years, finished his autobiography, was decorated by President & Mrs. Bush with the nation's highest civilian award, and left us two weeks later.

Unfortunately, too many of us did not learn to use our brains. Too many get the idea that the way to please their Creator is to grovel and humble themselves and be serious and sad. It has become a habit, a lifestyle. All of us have known people who are not happy unless they're miserable. Being miserable is a habit that is hard to break, and society gives us little reason to try. The reasons for breaking this negative habit, therefore, have to come from within each of us.

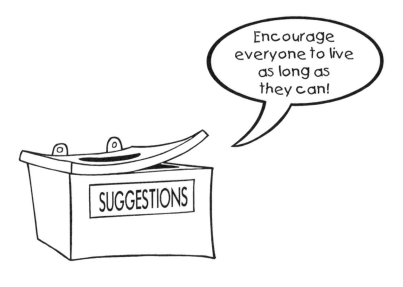

Full Speed Ahead!

It is time we quit feeling sorry for ourselves because of the mess we have made of our lives. We could have saved ourselves a lot of trouble if we had done a little thinking at the right time — **and Noah could have saved all of us a lot of misery if he had swatted those two flies**. Sure, we've made a lot of mistakes, but let's quit looking at the dark side and look at the bright. Only people who do something make mistakes, so we must have been doing an awfully lot to make so many. Maybe our heads swelled a little bit out of proportion, but so what? Let's learn from our mistakes and get back to work and having fun.

The present working generation has done as much to advance civilization as all the preceding generations. In other words, man has finally made a start in learning to think. Hallelujah! Hallelujah! One cannot help but wonder how happy our patient Creator must be. He is surely laughing or turning handsprings or whatever He does when He is thrilled. He waited a long time for us to start learning to use our marvelous brains. The entire history of our lack of use of this precious commodity can be recorded in only a few words: We were created as thinking humans, not robots, not slaves. This brain was given to us so that we could make our own decisions, and it put us in command of our lives, our own destiny. Our creator was so lavish in His gifts that he must have intended us to have fun, learn and grow, and be all that we can be. He wanted us to be assets, not liabilities, so that we could leave our world, His world, better than we found it. So He must be overjoyed that we are finally figuring out how to do just that.

Only recently I heard a story that explains it perfectly. It is about a man who prayed and prayed to win a lottery. Finally, he decided to ask the Lord why he had not won. The Lord replied, "George, give me a little help. Buy a lottery ticket." There are no freebies in life. Buy a ticket.

Sure, the last couple of generations have made some big mistakes in the midst of all this growth. But society is beginning to recognize the hangover with which it is waking up, and we are looking for some relief from the awful headache brought on by the drinking (spending) bout. We worked hard, became prosperous, decided to celebrate, cashed our pay checks, and got drunk. Our heads swelled; there wasn't a thing we could not do. The world was our oyster. We had reached the millennium. We enjoyed a long period of prosperity and happiness. We drank up our pay check, then gave the bartender IOU's. It took us nearly half a century to learn how to have glorious fun spending our grandchildren's money. We thought of Franklin Delano Roosevelt as our savior because he showed us how. But our big binge is almost over. It will not end, however, until we quit putting it "on the cuff" for our children and grandchildren to pay.

For decades we have seen our government on all levels become more crooked, costly, and arrogant and more and more our bosses. We have let the hired hand run the farm, and he is now the ruling class and has mortgaged the farm and pocketed the money. Our kids will look us in the eye and ask us why we let it happen. They resent it. They are already angry. "Granny Dumping" is on the rise as a result. Apparently, they do not like the heritage we are leaving them. They might not be quite so angry with us, though, if we can convince them that they, not us, will reap the most enjoyable benefits of our thinking and labor so they should help pay for it. We must help them find the positive side of their heritage —

> *we are leaving our children and grandchildren with all the information and technology they need to clean up our mess.*

While we accept and admit that we are human and prone to human mistakes, we can proudly explain that we knew we could not take this marvelous world with us, that we built it for them. Hopefully, they will buy that rationale. We have no other.

If our children and grandchildren even think of granny dumping us, we must tell them that, even though we're not proud of the $5 trillion debt we're leaving them, we can look them straight in the eye and unashamedly tell them that we made their world better than any other generation in history — and then challenge them to do as well.

So we have no need to feel guilty or to lash ourselves because we accomplished in 25 years as much as all the generations before ours. Our ancestors never made as big a mess because they didn't do as much thinking as we have done. We have proven that we are the best thinkers ever born so far.

Let us pat our own backs a bit, have some fun, and then turn this much better world we have created over to the next generation. Let's stop looking back when looking ahead is more fun. We cannot do anything about the past; it is history.

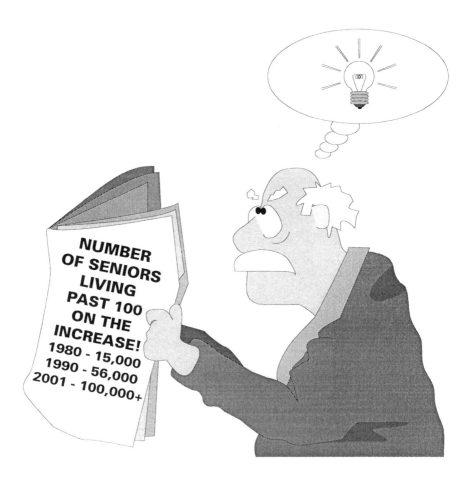

Look Forward, Seniors

Quit thinking that the odds are against you and saying that you never win anything because it's simply not true. In one race, where there were about 200 million entrants, you emerged as the winner. That was when you were conceived. You beat out 200 million others, so why turn chicken now when the odds are puny? Think of yourself as a winner, and you can be. That always comes first in any race.

Beginning at 60 and continuing until about 70, Seniors begin to divide into two groups. The 31% of Seniors who believe society's lies about aging are hoping to grow old in physical comfort while being afraid they will outlive their monetary resources. They let their brains die before they do and end up under the hill before they get past 75.

***If your brain dies, it is most
likely a do-it-yourself job.***

They number approximately two million each year. May they rest in peace. They leave us too early and take with them their experience and knowledge because they believe four lies.

- You're over the hill at sixty, and there's not much in life after that.
- You will live three score and ten years (70), the Biblical age.
- The rate of death goes up quite rapidly as you age. (No one tells you that that's only true until you reach 74, then it drops rapidly.
- Methuselah lived 970 years, but he was a freak. It will never happen again.

BALONEY!

- Those who were healthy at 60, who believed that over-the-hill-at-60 lie, were not told that those who followed it would be under the hill before they passed 75.
- The Bible gives us two choices as to how long we can live, 70 years or 120. Check Genesis 6:3 for "Man's life is one hundred and twenty years."
- For nearly 2,000 years, our Creator has been dangling that 970 like a carrot on a stick in front of us, hoping we would see it as a challenge to reach for 970. After all, Methuselah broke his grandfather's record by only four years, and it is the only unchallenged record in the world.

We cannot bring the 31% who dug their own graves back, but we can give ourselves a greater interest in life that will guarantee us many more and better tomorrows. We must learn how to do a better job of selling the negative thinkers among us on waking up and realizing that what 69% of us have already done can be done by anyone who tries. Even if only half that future 31% starts thinking positively, we will save a million a year of the best brains and experience to go on contributing to and participating in life. Saving a million people a year from a needlessly early grave will be a whale of an incentive for all of us in the 69% to go for 120 years of tomorrows in this wonderful world that is improving at a far faster rate than ever before.

The 69% who do their own thinking grew from 68% in 10 years between censuses. As these positive thinkers start over the hill, they begin picking up speed, fully intending to see how far they can go.

The facts are astounding. There will be two million people over the age of 90 by the end of this century. The number of people over 100 years of age more than tripled between 1980 and 1990. Actually, it was 363%. They now number approximately 56,000. It is predicted that there will be 100,000 by the end of this century — only four years down the road! And centenarians are not the only ones who have decided to live longer. In the period from 1980 to 1990, the number of 65 year olds increased 2%, and the number of 85 year olds increased 42%.

When I was born in 1899, I had a life expectancy of 37 years. Kids born today can expect about 75 (if they are not positive thinkers). At that rate of progress, every kid born in America will have a life expectancy of 969 years, Methuselah's age, by about the year AD 5379. Why wait 3300+ years?

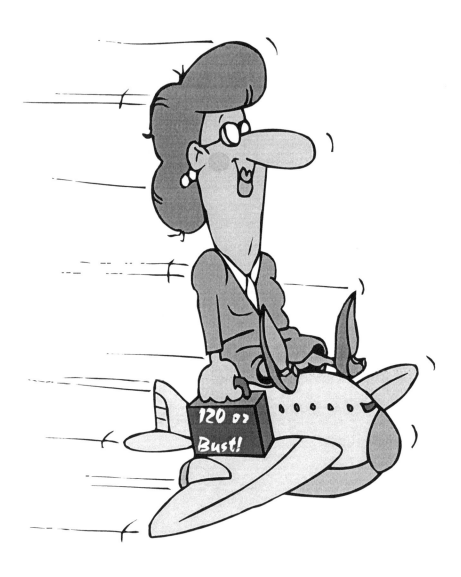

Change . . . It's a Positive Choice

Sometime after the wheel was invented but before we outran a horse, society's thinking about life was set in concrete. Most of its vast efforts, time, and money were working subtly toward one goal. Society has for generations been determined to help everyone grow old in physical comfort while paying no attention to whether the brain was kept alive and thriving, exactly the opposite of what it should have been doing. It should have been telling people to stay young, stay busy, have fun, and stay alive. As a result, 31% of all who reach 60 in good health do exactly as they are told to do: They go over the hill at 60 and under it before they can make it to 75.

The 69% who survive past 75, however, have done so because they have consciously or unconsciously chosen to ignore society's brainwashing and are still having fun while adding years and achievements to their lives. We are like the copper-top battery advertisements on TV — we keep going, and going, and going. Even though society knows that most people are on Cloud 9 the first few years in retirement, it has not given up, Even though more and more people are <u>choosing</u> to live longer, society in general just will not change its attitudes. Our bureaucrats know that doing the same thing over and over with the same people at the same place will put you in a rut and take some of the luster off retirement, and some retirees begin to wonder, "How long now?" Society doesn't give up.

Any time the question of age comes up, I ask, "How long do you expect to live?" Many are reluctant to answer. I get the feeling that they consider that the Lord's problem, not theirs. Quite a few say, "As long as I can," or words to that effect. They fall into the 69% positive thinking pile.

In 1988, I moved to Northwest Arkansas where at least half the people came from "up North" or California or Texas or Florida and are retired. I needed to study this problem society calls "aging." What I discovered is that most of society is traveling the wrong road toward the wrong goal. They remind me of the ancient joke about the two elk hunters who had just fired their last ammunition when a hungry grizzly saw them and started for them. One hunter pulled out his knife and started cutting off his heavy boots. The other, who was praying, stopped long enough to tell his friend, "You cannot outrun a bear." The man cutting off his boots replied, "I don't have to outrun that bear. All I have to do is outrun you."

It is fun to have neighbors who have succeeded and who are looking ahead to more of the harvest time of life. You occasionally find one, though, who has fallen in love with and practices negative living, but you must not let him bother you because he is not long for this world. You realize that it makes much more sense to look ahead to the bright side of everything, so you seek the company of the neighbors who have found another Santa. They make the best neighbors.

Choosing not to make changes for yourself to get you out of any rut will cause you to seek the old rocking chair more and more, and the undertakers will soon be telling your grieving family and friends that they were fortunate to have had you for so long. This is what happens when you retire and believe you are over the hill. So don't sit in that rocker (the greatest killing machine ever invented) comparing your aches and pains and arthritis and heart trouble and irregularity and miseries and looking for the dark side of everything with all your friends. Get up and join the rest of us who are intent on making the 50 years after 70 the best of our lives.

People, honeybees, and buzzards generally find what they look for.

Seniors who are caught in the cycle of negative thinking that makes them believe they are over the hill and useless need to make some changes. They need to get something new — a new car, a new hobby, a new wife or husband — or they will begin to really believe that retirement is just a place to wait for the undertaker. Most people who let their brains die before their bodies do are merely obeying what they have been taught by our well-meaning society, that loss of mental ability is a part of the aging process and is to be expected. **BULL!** The Seniors who live the longest are the ones who continue to use their brains. If you doubt it, make a list of your friends who have died. Also make a list of those who are expecting to die. The ones who do the most thinking and look forward to each day as a new adventure and opportunity to learn or find something new to be excited about in both groups will be the survivors. The ones on your lists who begin to

wonder, "How long?" will depart first. Those who contribute to the world about them find reasons to prolong and
enjoy their lives. Those who contribute nothing to their
world become spectators, and there isn't a whole lot of
room for spectators in retirement. The idea of staying
young and having fun and the idea of growing old are as
different as a nursery and a mortuary.

There ain't no stress in retirement. There are no
alarm clocks. You can roll over and go back to sleep all
day, but you will not. You will sleep just long enough to
enjoy the feeling that you can do it. You can do exactly as
you please, when you please. You can loaf, or you can
work if you want to, and you can quit when you want to.
You are the boss, the King of the Mountain. You are in
command, the master of your fate. You can mope and feel
sorry for yourself, or you can have fun and enjoy life. The
decision is strictly yours. You can wonder how long
you're going to live, or you can really live. You can sit and
wait for the undertaker, or you can have fun helping others not
so fortunate as you. It is popular because it feeds our egos by
making us proud, and being proud keeps us young.

Most Seniors expect to rest and enjoy life for a few
years after retirement, but far too many drift aimlessly
through retirement not knowing how long it will be before
the fat lady sings and without knowing where they're
going. Unfortunately, many don't realize they need to go
anywhere. It's hard enough to get anywhere when you
don't know your destination, but it's downright impossible
to get anywhere when there's not even a thought of making
a journey. At first, many retirees follow their hobbies from
daylight to dark, and too many never learn that a life of
self-satisfying golf or other hobby is not a full life. Some
retirees do volunteer work.

Every community has groups organized to find opportunities for people who want to help others, and they can offer you a long list of jobs that need doing. If you happen to be in the rare community that doesn't have a volunteer group like this, start one yourself. You will be amazed and delighted when you discover how many things need to be done that only your special talent or personality can accomplish. Perhaps you are THE one to start this type of activity for the betterment of your own community and the extended years it will bring you and your peers. You can become the hub of an entirely new and beneficial outreach program that will touch many lives in your own community. I knew a lady who worked two afternoons a week in a hospital gift shop. At 96+, she was making plans for her 100th birthday. This is but one example of what positive thinking — and action — can do for all retirees.

Even though we have seen others do it and live long lives, far too many of us never grasp that just setting a goal would brighten the way and enable us to plan for more fun or that there is untold fun to be had by helping others live longer lives.

Too many of us believe funeral dates are set by God, completely overlooking the fact that God gave us a brain so that we can make our own decisions.

Why would He give us these wonderful brains if He intended to guide every step we take? He could have built an army of robots easier and with less emotional hassles. Does God expect to baby sit us through our lives? All parents with grown kids know there came a time when they were READY for their offspring to fly the coop. Why wouldn't God want us to fly with our own wings? Those who say they are afraid to step on the Lord's toes by setting their own goals for the length of their lives are simply refusing to take responsibility for themselves and blaming the Lord for an early departure. In my opinion, those who refuse to use their brains are the ones stepping on the Lord's heart.

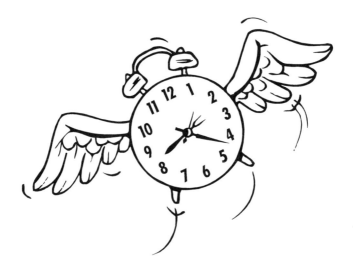

One of life's indisputable truths is that time also flies when you're not having fun.

Positive Breeds Positive

Our length of life is set by our mental attitude. If we think we can survive happily and productively, we do. Everyone has to feel needed, but no one can feel needed unless they are of some use to someone. Staying alive just to show grandchildren they can is a reason used by many. Some volunteer for menial tasks, but it matters little whether the work is considered menial. I knew a woman years ago who went camping frequently with a group on weekends. She had given $2100 to a Seeing Eye Dog foundation by picking up aluminum cans around camp-grounds and roads nearby. Others reach for their handful of stars by stimulating public interest in various causes; some serve quietly, some more loudly. All are valuable. All are needed for the health of our entire society. All work is honorable.

It is hard to believe that many retirees cannot find what to do with their spare time. Of course, many of them have never had enough spare time to learn how to handle it. They are not prepared for retirement. The builder and operator of a successful business is treated as if he is senile the day after he retires, so he is left out of conversations and plans — even the ones being made for him. "Helpers" begin to indulge him more and more because of his "increasing deterioration." This builder, this successful thinking man makes an unconscious decision to allow himself to become almost a vegetable. What a waste! Especially when there so many opportunities for him to use his vast knowledge and abilities that would extend his life and create a better world for everyone.

Some Seniors begin retirement with hobbies like golf, hobbies that lose some luster in anywhere from one to thirty years. Fishing ends when you cannot look a fish in the face anymore. That can happen in two weeks or fifty years, and apparently, bridge outlasts all other hobbies. (One lady I knew quit at 97 when we buried her.)

The biggest mistake any retiree can make is to think, "Now I've got it made. I can rest and do as I please as I've dreamed for years." They quit learning and growing and begin to die, but do not realize it. They think that when they quit working, the world quits changing and growing, too. They make new friends and drift along in a state of bliss for a few years. Gradually, they get a belly full of their hobbies, no longer as attractive as they were. Unconsciously, the choosing begins, and retirees either opt for the rocking chair or begin exploring avenues to be productive. They know they still owe civic duties of some kind, so they volunteer for various charities at least half a day a week, and often much more. The positive-thinking retirees find that volunteering to help others gradually begins to cut down on hobby time, and they learn that self-recreation is by no means a full life.

A small percentage of retirees do a lot of reading. Too often, though, they read just the local paper to see what their neighbors are doing. News about what is going on in the outside world is provided by television, but the negative-thinking retirees are not as interested in it as they should be. They are inclined to think that the world quit changing when they retired. Very, very few read books. Many seem to believe that the status quo will last for their lifetimes.

A surprising number of retirees simply go back to work. Sometimes it is the old job, but more often, it is an entirely new career. Even more surprising is that many of these new careers are more exciting, satisfying, and lucrative than the ones from which they retired. Why not? How many of you stayed in jobs you were not entirely delighted with because of economics, educational requirements, etc., and always dreamed of working in another profession? Now you can do whatever it was you always thought you wanted to do. Now is the time you can spread your wings. Now you can go back to school if need be, invent that thingamajig that every human being needs that will only cost a dollar, start your own home business creating greeting cards — **WHATEVER!!** You can do it now!

When hobbies lose their allure, the old rocking chair creeps into the picture and begins competing for our time and interest. If it wins, so does the undertaker's pocketbook. Those who begin volunteering more and helping others more find their lives richly rewarded, so they like it here and intend to stay. If doubling or quadrupling or changing the nature of the volunteer work you do doesn't seem to be working for you, go look at the tombstones of the last three friends your age who let boredom and feeling sorry for themselves take them away. Surely you can have more fun than they and make a contribution in the process.

Heaven can wait for you, and so can the undertaker.

My kid brother kept very busy tending a garden about 20 feet long and 10 feet wide. It kept him and his brain alive until he was 85. As I remember him, he got more joy out of his ailments than most people.

A hobby that can give you an interest in life is to write a book describing all the changes you have seen in your lifetime. It may not have any present value, but it will be priceless to your grandchildren and their children, and it is really quite fun. I wrote one for a nephew. Kids today get a bang out of it because things have changed so much.

A possible new hobby to explore would be to gain more understanding of ESP (extra sensory perception). We have known of its existence for centuries, but we have learned very little about it. Lots of people have a little of it. I know a lady who sells mostly Bibles and religious cards. She claims she can recognize a Methodist and one other denomination the minute they walk into her store. I told her that I believe her. I have the ability to feel in the first few seconds of meeting a person if that person thinks that a 96-year-old person has been overlooked by the undertaker for 26 years. If so, I have some fun. I try to work into a position so I can tell him I am coming to his funeral.

There are probably hundreds of examples like the above. The more we use our brains, the longer we will live and have fun. Why not try to solve the problems that confront us daily? Recently I had to learn childproof bottles can be opened with one hand. My right hand was in a cast because of a broken bone. It took me 3 hours and 35 minutes to get my medicine, but I got it — without whining about the injustices of the pharmaceutical companies or bothering someone else to do what I could do for myself. Until faced with a dilemma to work through, I often couldn't open those pesky bottles with both hands! I feel so proud that now I have a new hobby and am looking for answers to all questions. It helps me stay young.

We must all nurture the will to live. The best description of how this will to live works is that of a famous dog. His right ear was missing, he was blind in his left eye, his left paw could not reach the ground, and he had castrated himself jumping a barbed wire fence, but he still answered to the name of Lucky. That's about the most positive attitude I've ever come across, but I think it shows how precious all our lives are even though we may have some artificial parts and the original parts don't work quite as well as they used to.

Retirees who stay busy and cleanse their minds of negative trash the quickest live the longest. The better you clear your mind, the happier you will be and the longer you will live.

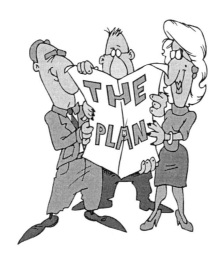

Don't snicker at the words "second childhood" because it can actually be better and last a lot longer than the first one — which ended when you were told that there ain't no Santa Claus. Its only weakness is that you cannot open child-proof medicine bottles. You still have to get your grandchildren to do that.

Second childhood can begin after 74 and last another 40+ years. It is better because by 74, or soon after, you are as smart as you thought you were at 17. You know what is important and what is not, what is worth fighting for and what to forget. You know what to expect in life and how to get it. You have the tools to plan to get the most out of life. You are more serene. Your vision is better though your eyesight may be dimmer.

Somewhere along the line, if you want to live as long as you can, you must choose to become a positive thinker whose choice is not to join the 31% who believe they have an obligation to die before 75. You continue learning and looking forward to each new day or you know you won't stay here. You are traveling the right road to a successful, long life and plan to die young at whatever age, including 970 years.

George Burns is an example that proves that the second childhood is better and longer than the first. George said the he couldn't help growing old, but that he was not going to get OLD. What he meant is that as the years pass, his body may slow down physically, but he never will. He did not let his brain die from lack of use. Many thought his words just a joke, but George knew that just setting a goal gives everyone an interest in life that helps keep people alive and young. He also knew that this kind of attitude brightens the road ahead.

George Burns probably didn't have an enemy in the world. Why is that? He was a positive thinking role model, always looking ahead. His happy outlook rubbed off on everyone because just looking at him gave everyone a lift. Just mentioning his name brings a smile to every-one. What a wonderful legacy to leave with us. It would surely be a more joyous world if everyone tried to imitate George, that is something all of us are capable of doing. George was just himself. He was in command of George, just as you are of your life. He had no magic wand to wave to produce the results he wanted. He needed none. He was just an ordinary mortal who never stopped growing men-tally. After years of practice, getting smarter and happier every year, of course he outshone most of us. But George was one of those people who never questioned if he could or not — he just did it, whatever it was.

Bob Hope survived his 90th birthday party where the whole world made it very plain that they thought he had come to the end of the line and they never expected to wish him another happy birthday. A great many wished him a happy birthday, but only five or six added, "and many happy returns." Obviously, most thought it his last. That is how our lives are shortened. Hope's friends meant no harm. Far from it. They were merely playing the role that all Seniors play in helping one another grow old. They haven't even questioned the idea that no one has to grow old, so they become unconscious conspirators in early funerals.

I have done more thinking after 90 than I did in the 90 years before. It was fun figuring out why people die at an average age of 74 and why women outlive men. I can see a lot of our problems more clearly now and that most have a simple solution. As Shad Helmstetter told us, "Nothing is more impossible than you think it is." Ziggy Ziglar tells us, "What you put in your mind, you are." The Bible says, "As a man thinketh, so is he."

At 96, I am planning to go to 120 and have more fun every year than the year before. Of course, I know that I may not make it all the way, but I also know that each year I do have will be more fun than the one before. I have my third pacemaker, and if it quits, so will I. I waste no time thinking about death. Why should I? Death has three bright sides (to a positive thinker): I do not have to die but once. My troubles will be over. I'm going to a better home. I cannot lose by going for 120, and I will have more fun than if I had not tried. When I do die, I do not expect to take anything with me. Whatever I build, big or small, I will try to leave in the best hands possible.

I think better now than ever before. I am better equipped than ever before. I always look for the bright side and avoid all negative thinking. Many of my aches and pains have gone away. For most of us, they are not in our joints anyway; they are between our ears and easily cured.

I have learned, after lots of practice, that there are only two ways to reduce the pain of troubles. Troubles have minds of their own. They pick on people who will pay them the most attention. I can deflate their egos and pull their fangs by ignoring them or by laughing at them. They may not go away, but they are less painful and easier to live with. It makes them realize that I am still in command of myself and my attitude. You must remember to never, never, never let anything or anyone get you down. You are in command.

After you are 74, when you are told something, you are more likely to use your brain and examine it. You make your own decisions as to true or false. You know that you got to 74 and are still going because you learned to look for the bright, the positive side. You are very aware that the friends and family you have lost unwittingly looked for the dark side — and found it. When they spoke of some coming event, they usually prefaced their opinion or decision with, "If I am still alive and am able, I will do so and so." Or worse yet, they often said, "God willing, I will do the following." They forget that God gave His consent when He gave us brains so we could make our own decisions.

It is easy to understand why anyone born before 1950 would tend to follow in his father's mental footsteps. The world used to change slowly. I remember getting a child's knife, fork, and spoon in a little white-cardboard, purple-lined box while sitting in a high chair at the table. My siblings, years later, insisted it was my eighth birthday. My next memory was toddling with my mother holding my hand past an open door of a store called Nickelodeon and seeing motion pictures on a screen at the back of the store. The stores of that era had changed hardly at all 25 years later. Today, stores of all kinds change more in one year than in the 25 at the beginning of this century. The later after 1950 a person was born, the less excuse he has for cobwebs between his ears.

You cannot stay young by letting the world pass you by. You have to keep up with it, and you can stay ahead of it if you try.

You have the advantage of experience. You do not have to become a convert to every fool idea that comes along. I have managed to get by without rock and roll and the later, noisier varieties of music. I did make the mistake of smoking a pipe for 30 years, but I quit instantly in 1952. Another mistake I made was to wear jockey shorts or briefs until a Dear Abby column warned me of their effect. Her column was correct.

My point is that you can pick and choose the new ideas and gadgets that suit you and that you want to use. Be aware of the ones you do not like and make sure they do not hurt you, then let them go their way. From 74 on, the things you learned in the boot camp of life can guide you wisely. Put your experience to work to live life to its fullest. That is why that half century after 70 was given to you.

The Dawning

I must have believed the over-the-hill lie at some point. In 1987, I was driving to St. Louis to attend a convention of Quiet Birdmen and stopped to see an old friend. His greeting was, "Have you bought any new shoes?" I asked what he was talking about, and he laughed and reminded me that in 1962, he had thought to do me a favor by telling me of a going-out-of-business sale at a nearby shoe store where I could load up on shoes at bargain prices. I told him, "No, thanks. I am pretty sure I have all the shoes I will ever need." When I think of how full and happy my life is at 96, it's hard for even me to believe I never expected to get past 70. Christmas cards from my friend always say, "Another year, another pair of shoes."

I was surprised at about 70, however, to find myself unburied, in good health, enjoying life, and I was not anywhere over the hill. My prime was ahead of me several years. I had been had, and that's when I realized that society had lied to me about old age, so I began looking at everything else I had been taught and questioning the truthfulness of all the preconceived notions about growing old. Since I knew that liars never tell just one lie, I began looking for others, and it soon became apparent that much of what society had been feeding me was false. The centuries-old dread of "growing OLD" that has soured the lives of untold millions and sent them to early graves is no longer true, if it ever was. The people themselves are beginning to bury that negative thinking and are switching to the bright side, positive thinking, and happier, longer lives. My fault in the "scheme" was that I chose for far too many years to believe.

At some point, however, I began wondering if I could possibly make it to 83, as my dad did. Was that my prerogative or God's? Friends I asked seemed embarrassed and afraid to even talk about it. They were afraid they would be stepping on the Lord's toes. I thought it over for months. Finally, I realized God had given me a brain, so he must have expected me to use it and make my own decisions. I decided that when He gave me a brain, He put me in command of my own destiny. He wanted to see if I could live and grow and become an asset and help Him in making a better world.

I began to wonder if all the great minds in society were overlooking something. I remembered that back in the mid-thirties, a Professor Goddard in Massachusetts had seen a potential in rockets that no one else had seen, though the Chinese invented them three thousand years before. He did a lot of experimenting on them and successfully launched what was then a super rocket. He told people he thought they could carry mail. What he really had in mind was to sell the idea to the Army, but our Army was not interested. Neither was any other army. But a screwball in Germany must have read the papers because a few years later, he acquired Goddard's data and equations and built a V1 and a V2 rocket and destroyed a lot of

London. His name was Hitler. He was the only man in the world to see the potential, but after he showed us what could be done with the technology, we took over and developed it further. We carried on where he left off, and 12 Americans have walked on the moon, and we are now working on a manned, nuclear-powered space rocket to put men on Mars. We have a probe traveling 40,000 miles per hour exploring the universe some 18 billion miles from Earth. Perhaps the only positive title that could be bestowed on Hitler is "Father of Space Travel."

Today, when I see pictures of men walking on the moon and pictures of several planets sent back by cameras roaming the nearby universe, I am impressed. I remember the billions and billions of stars and the Milky Way that I saw clearly as a youngster but are no longer visible due to air pollution.

It has been a lot of years since I have seen more than a dozen or so stars in the sky, but my recollection of them and their impression on me is as vivid as ever. I get the same feeling today by going into the woods and watching the mighty forces of Nature at work, the trees competing for sunlight, every living thing engaged in the law of survival of the fittest. It's a feeling not found in churches. I am fascinated and awed by the enormity of it. Then I read that we are building more powerful telescopes so we can see an even more vast universe that is out there, but we still cannot see it. Whoever created it sure had a busy week. He can be proud. One wonders what in it He is most proud of. My guess is that He would pick the human brain as His masterpiece of creation.

I make no pretense of being what is generally considered religious. What little I acquired was done so while sitting on the back porch of our farm home with the family looking to the east as the stars and the Milky Way were hung in the sky after the sun went down. I probably asked who hung them there. I was told that an all-powerful person called God had created them and the world and us and everything else. Mother pointed out the Big Dipper and the Little Dipper and some other stars that had names. I'm sure that show is staged every evening, but I have not seen it in years.

My parents talked of God with respect but no fear. I believe they felt that anyone so powerful was not afraid of them and saw no reason to fear Him. They told me that all I need do was treat others as I expected to be treated and I had nothing to fear either. It has worked for me and will not be changed. It is the best religion I have encountered. If there is any more to religion than that, I have not found it nor am I looking for it. If I were interested in finding more to religion, I might examine some of the things the holy men tell me I must do to get into Heaven.

Somehow, I know my Creator is not angry because I have postponed my funeral. He has postponed it for me himself half a dozen times in my long, full life.

The Stay Young Land

I have studied what I call the "Stay Young Land" since 1985, when its place in the Universe first dawned on me. It is that little piece of the territory in a person's life that can only be explored after you go beyond the 74th year cemetery fence. Ponce de Leon wandered the Earth for years looking for the fountain of youth. He never found it. We have. It's right between our own ears, and we are beginning to explore ways to enjoy and improve this Stay Young Land for ourselves and anyone else who chooses to join us. Now that we know what it is and where it is, we will advertise its location.

I must be the luckiest retiree in the world. So many retirees have trouble finding something to do to give them an interest in life. Why not join me in exploring this new area and telling those who are still here with us but aren't sure why that this can be their home until they are 120. I believe we can convince at least half those who die before 75 to join us and continue the Great Easter Egg Hunt to find more goodies our Creator left for us. As Gil Robb Wilson said, "Flying wings are not for those who are content with pottage."

When you graduate from the life's boot camp into retirement, you can give yourself a wonderful second chance by realizing that it is not the end of anything except the frustrations and stresses of raising a family and making a living. It is a commencement program like those from high school or college. It is a reincarnation, the beginning of a new life, but it is a life in which you will not make the same youthful mistakes again. You know your own abilities and have proved them once and know you can do even better the second time. You do not have to waste time experimenting and feeling your way before doing something. It would be a shame to junk all your hard-earned knowledge and experience. You are a part of our country's — no, the world's greatest asset: the experience of our Senior citizens.

You don't have to pack away any of your knowledge or experience. There are a multitude of ways you can once again show the world that you are still alive and a proud and contributing part of it.

Our world is not and never has been a daycare center for weaklings. One of God's paramount rules of the natural world is survival of the fittest. It governs every living thing on earth, and no attempt to amend it will ever succeed. It is a just law. It always grieves me to hear anyone ask their Creator to guide every step they take. They must think of him as their baby sitter. They have twisted the Bible statement that says He created man in His own image to "God was created in man's image, pin head and all." I repeat, we were created as humans, not slaves and not robots.

Just Look Around

"Physically J am failing: my sense, my locomo-
tive powers, my memory are decaying . . . yet my
mind feels capable of growth; for my curiosity is
keener than ever . . . J might begin a political
career as a junior civil servant and evolve into a
Cabinet minister in another hundred years or so."

—George Bernard Shaw
Back to Methuselah

Just walk into a Wal-Mart store or grocery store or
hardware store once a month and look at the new goodies
that were not there the month before. You will soon begin to
realize what man's learning to think has accomplished. When
we are told that half the knowledge we have accumulated
since time began has been discovered in the last 25 years, we
begin to feel the speed of change that thinking has brought
about. Thinking has caused an avalanche of material goodies
for us to enjoy, and they are all welcome. It is time to recognize, however, that the greatest source of all this luxury is
beginning to come from between our own ears.

Most of the advances we have enjoyed since we outran a horse in 1829 have been technical in nature — improved and newly invented tools, machinery, etc. Now, both plants and animals are being upgraded or are being genetically engineered and improved or are making it to the market for the first time. Strange fruits and vegetables you've never heard of are offered in the markets today. Many fruits and vegetables we could only read about and see pictures of not too far back are in abundance on the shelves of most of our stores year around, and there is little need to think about what is "in season" at any given time. Technology, man's ingenuity.

Even we humans are today being eyed for improvement by science. Why not? Some of us are less than perfect. And don't worry about improving our Creator's product. He will be proud and delighted to see us improve on his masterpiece. I believe He will be our most enthusiastic booster. Remember, He's the one who gave us these thinking brains. If we use our brains to improve ourselves, like we do with animals and plants, He will realize His gift of a brain was not a waste of time.

We have known for a long, long time that there is a very fine line between genius and insanity. My mother used to joke by telling people that she never had worried about any of her six kids going insane — that none of them were smart enough. I don't know about the my five siblings, but that made me realize that my mother, who could read and write and add two plus two and get four, was no dummy. She had little education, but plenty of common sense. Always, when I have met a few people I was told were off their rockers, I have realized that their wildest ideas may look crazy to us, but that may be due to our being dumb and that some of it may be too smart for us to understand. I will not be surprised to find investigators being accused of being insane. They will be the ones who learn. We think we know how normal brains work. The only way to improve our performance is to study how <u>all</u> brains work, including those of the insane. They are quite possibly the most promising field to study.

Roger Bannister's four-minute mile and Sputnik came almost at the same time. Which will benefit humanity more, the Space Age or the exploration of another small part of the human brain? The only thing we know now is the inspiration both gave us. Who knows? Exploring that part of the brain that controls mental attitude may be of bigger benefit to humanity than unlocking the secrets of the atom.

What a wonderful world this will be when we spend as much time exploring our own brains as we do on technological improvements.

Undoubtedly, improvement in our brains will make us happier than any amount of technical progress. All we have to do to make our mental improvement exceed our technical improvements is to switch our thinking from three-quarters negative to positive. Nothing is ever done until someone thinks it can be done, and then works at it until he finds out how.

Our brains have amply demonstrated their ability to improve technical things. Isn't it about time to devote a big share of that ability to developing the human mind to improve human relations as much as we have the technical? It will be embarrassing to land men with Julius Caesar-era brains on Mars. Let's cut out the negative thinking — always looking on the dark side — and develop our brains to fit into the Space Age. It can be easier and much more rewarding than the technical development.

Work is being done now on making the learning process faster and more simple. I wish I had had some of these wonderful opportunities when I was in the third grade. Young people today take for granted concepts that we weren't even introduced to until we were nearing adulthood. Yet, it is necessary that we all remember that it was our generation that brought so much of what we all enjoy today to fruition — without all this scientific knowledge.

Little by little, we discover minute scraps of information about mental attitude that amaze us. Isn't it time we make a conscious, planned effort to explore the last frontier: our own minds? I suspect that "We ain't seen nothin' yet." Exploring the uncharted territory between our ears will probably look like the dawn of civilization in a generation or two. Exploring where no man has gone before is immensely rewarding.

Unfortunately, on the subject of aging, our society is still in the horse and buggy era.

Negative Thinking Breeds Bureaucracies

How did those of us who have lived beyond our life expectancy do it? Positive thinking. That is the sole reason, and it is sufficient. So why, then, hasn't society in general jumped on our bandwagon and started looking at a more positive way of "dealing" with us? The reason is quite plain when you think about it. We all dislike change. Society hates change even more than individuals because it is composed almost entirely of hundreds of big and little bureaucracies. The private ones are worse than the government ones. Theoretically, government bureaucracies have to answer to the voters. All bureaucracies are political machines just like courthouses. Dealing with any of them is like dealing with the government.

Trade organizations, clubs of all kinds, unions, churches, charities, etc., are usually mini-bureaucracies, and it is time we began looking at them. United Way had the same head man for 22 years, at a salary of over $400,000 a year. Another big charity changes presidents every two years. Capable businessmen fight for the job and work for no pay. They do not need pay, nor do they need to steal if they can spend the budget in the right places. There are lots of ways where a not-for-profit organization is smarter than one for profit.

Let's take a look at one charity group. There are approximately 378 organizations engaged in whole organ transplants. (The 65 organizations working on eyesight problems and sight for the blind are not included in this examination.) In 1991, 300 experts met for a two-day seminar at the University of Michigan to discuss ways to get more people to donate organs. In the preceding year, they had found 4500 donors who donated 15,000 organs that were transplanted. They even discussed buying organs.

I read about the seminar in the *Arkansas Democrat*, and about lunchtime on the second day, I called the lady who had charge of arranging the seminar. I told her that I had a sales talk of about 40 words that I had used for about 3 minutes at the close of each of my speeches that had signed up over 25% of many audiences to donate corneas and two-thirds had donated organs as well. An average of 25% is a whole lot better than one out of 600,000 people, as the so-called experts had done. I gave her the exact number of donors I had filed at the state-owned Eye Bank and Laboratory in Little Rock and gave her the phone number so she could check my veracity, then tell the experts at their afternoon meeting how I had succeeded in doing that. She refused.

The next day, I wrote her a letter. No reply to date. I quit speaking to write this book. My count to date is 358 eye donor cards, two-thirds of which also donated organs. It took three minutes at the close of 18 speeches — about one hour of selling time. This is the sales talk:

"If you were St. Peter, guarding the gate to Heaven, and two people arrived with equal qualifications, except one was an eye and organ donor and the other was not, which one would you let in if you had room for only one?"

Let's find out what is wrong. Surely, more than one American in 600,000 would be willing to part with things they have no further use for.

Bureaucrats are people. They protect one another (unless they can steal a job), and they cover up for one another. Their jobs are often more secure than political jobs or private ones. All of them resist change; they would have to learn something new. Most have a bit of Puritan blood in them. Puritans are people who cannot sleep at night. They are afraid that somewhere, somehow, someone will be having a good time. People who have a good time are often boat rockers, and bureaucrats are always on guard against boat rockers. People who think for themselves and question the status quo are always capable of rocking boats.

Nuclear bombs are not powerful enough to blast society out of its set-in-concrete, horse-and-buggy, negative and depressing thinking about aging. The thing that can and will do it is a positive mental attitude put forth by all of us Seniors every day of our lives in all our dealings with them. The 69% of us who escape the undertaker at around 74 are treated as freaks, not as role models, by our society. We do not mind. We are having far more fun than the 31% who chose to lay down at the bottom of the first hill instead of continuing to climb up another.

Everyone is living longer now, and the segment of population above 85 is the fastest growing. In 1980, there were 15,000 centenarians. By 1990, there were 56,000, more than three and a half times as many. When Willard Scott congratulates people on their 100th birthday on TV, others are probably persuaded to go for 100. The most noticeable thing about Mr. Scott's congratulations is that the number of people who are 105, 108, 110 or more is increasing. When the program first started, very, very few ever reached 101 or more. Apparently, the goal had been 100, and when that was reached, the people knew of no reason to go on living and believed they had come to the end of their road — therefore, it was. If Mr. Scott would encourage people to go for 110 or 120, many would do it. Along with his recognition of these centenarians, he could point out that they are role models and urge them to do humanity an even bigger favor than they have already by going for 120 as their Bible says they can. He might be very pleasantly surprised to find how little urging is needed, and in the process, he would be programming himself to do the same. A real win-win situation for everyone since a centenarian is no more likely to die than he was at 74.

If death is impending, people fight to live. If it is in the future, they go on smoking.

Everyone fights fiercely against immediate death. If the danger is not immediate, it is not feared. That is why persuading people to live longer is such a hard job. If a hungry lion were turned loose in your neighborhood, you would instantly arrange for protection.

Humans pay too little attention to other slow killers like cigarettes, booze, drugs, obesity, and on the greatest killer of all, negative thinking. It is not even recognized as a killer, but it kills 31% of all who reach 60 in good health within 14 years of their 60th birthdays. Over two million Americans a year go that route.

Some may ask, "What good are these centenarians?" It is true that many of them are not mental giants or great performers. They do, however, earn their keep. Their ability to survive holds out hope for all of us to do as well. Hope is precious. Let's study how they do it.

Obviously, they long ago quit thinking 85 or 95 was OLD and now realize it is not years that make you old, but thinking you are old will do it. Most of life's problems have simple answers. Quit thinking about getting OLD. Think instead of staying young, and you will.

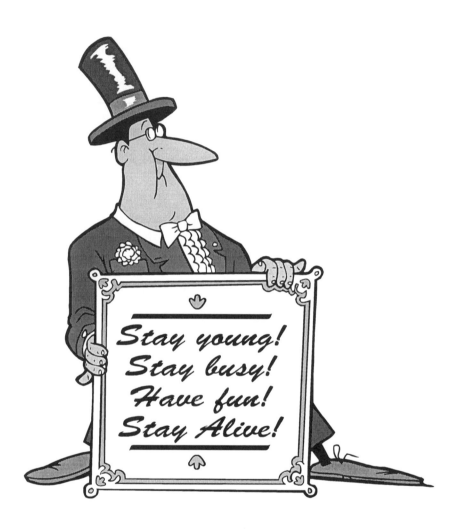

It Really Does Cost Nothing

We human beings are funny people. We are born into the world as positive thinkers, and then we proceed to turn much of our positive thinking into negative. Every child looks forward to happy events like Christmas and birthdays. Even children who have been repeatedly disappointed anticipate what they just somehow know are supposed to be happy events in their lives. For our first five years, most of us are gloriously happy.

When we are around five, however, those who run our schools, churches, charities, and all of society's government impress upon us their first lie — they tell us that there ain't no Santa Claus. Now, those of us who choose to live beyond 75 **KNOW** there will always be a Santa Claus. We know he is still making his rounds and that those little kids we used to be are still alive in our hearts. Listen to those little kids and be happy again. It works for grownups, too. Think of your glass as half full, not as half empty, and smile instead of frowning. The sun will surely shine if you do. Being happy or miserable cost the same — nothing, but the end results are vastly different.

Your happiness and your misery are controlled by your own mental attitude. Controlling it is not a very big job, and it requires less work to be happy than to be miserable. So why isn't everyone gloriously happy all the time? Let's think through to the answer.

A small minority of people do not want to be happy as we know happiness. The nearest they ever come to being happy is when they are downright miserable. Depriving them of their suffering would ruin their day. We all have met such people. We tend to feel sorry for them even though we know our compassion is being wasted. We would get no thanks if we tried to help them. What they want to do with their lives is their business, not ours. All we can do is to be ready to help them if and when they start using their own brains and recognize their own control over their lives. Our time and energies are better spent where we can get positive, lasting results. (We all know lots of people who rarely use their brains. Of course, those of us who have observed this fault in others rarely look into mirrors.)

We positive thinkers have chosen not to believe we are over the hill at 60 or that there is not much left in life after 65 or that we should enjoy what we can of our lives waiting for the inevitable at three score and ten (70 years). We are told that is the life span of man as revealed in the Bible, but there is no mention made of Genesis 6:3 which says: "Man's life is 120 years." Some Bible scholars tell us that the Lord simply changed his mind later on, or they simply disagree. I was told one time that there was a string attached to that 120 years. Whether that "string" is one man's interpretation or God's, I do not know. I do know, however, that our spiritual leaders have kept Genesis 6:3 in the closet.

It is not religion that has let us down. It is not just a case of the blind leading the blind. It is human frailty. Our spiritual leaders overlook the abilities and the tools and the intelligence and the choices our Creator gave us. I truly believe these gifts were given to us because He hoped we would grow and be all that we could be. Only then would we be able to do a good job of what He put us here to do: make our world a little better.

All of the El Toro Poo Poo is effective. Too many of us are switched from our positive thinking child to negative thinking retirees. By the time we are ready to retire, about three-fourths of our thinking has become negative. We stop thinking we can be vital, contributing members of society; therefore, too many of us aren't.

Methuselah lived 969 years (without "help"), and it most likely had more to do with the quality of his life than the years piled up. We are told that this is a freak of nature, like two heads, and is not supposed to happen. BA-LONEY! Methuselah's dad lived 365 years and his granddad lived 965. Both are rarely mentioned. Methuselah broke his grandfather's record by only four years. The Lord could not have made it any more plain that He would be pleased to welcome a new champion, and we humans are notorious for wanting to break records.

Another glorious picker upper that is still kept in the closet is that the number of deaths per 1000 increases rapidly to the age of 74. Several times as many 74 years olds per 1000 die as 60 year olds. After 74, it starts decreasing. At 96, my chance of living another year are slightly better than 97%. The road has leveled out. If society "trained" us to believe these facts instead of the lies and myths they obviously feel compelled to perpetuate, more of us might opt to live that extra half century beyond 70.

Methuselah — is it possible that he lived to such a long life because he didn't have so much "help" in his "old age" that he failed? If he came back today to set a new record, he would find three enormous roadblocks that have evolved in our society that pave the road to the landfill (also known as "cemetery") for many of us. It would be interesting to see his reaction to all of the well-meaning, kind-hearted doctors, social workers, religious leaders, bureaucrats, and, yes, even family members who would insist on helping him to GROW OLD. These genuinely well-meaning folks unwittingly perpetuate the myths of how retirement and "old age" are supposed to be because they themselves believe them. They pride themselves on their work in helping Seniors grow old in physical comfort. They think they are being kind when they coddle Seniors into thinking they need help while growing old. Growing old is the only thing on their minds. They consider it universal and inevitable.

Methuselah would surely be amazed when he ran into the next road block and found literally millions of volunteer do gooders, reinforced by 9,000 Senior Citizen Centers run by paid bureaucrats making a career out of seeing to it that Seniors know they need help and should come to the center and play dominoes while their brains die. In convincing retirees of this, they protect their jobs. They work in nice offices and have lots of staff members and a nice fleet of station wagons in the parking lot. How much of the budget do the Seniors actually see? I don't know. I would hope for at least 25%. But imagine paying people to help you grow old. How silly can we get? Why not pay them for helping us stay young? My guess is that there are few Seniors who are not given the opportunity and some coaxing to become dependent on these bureaucracies.

The third road block Methuselah would find is about 670 area Agencies on Aging across the country. Nine are in the small state of Arkansas. In 1994, the one in Fort Smith, Arkansas, had 950 employees who made 134,000 house calls on Seniors at a cost of $13 million — about $100 per visit. I have foregone the research to find the figures for what all the other agencies cost, but 670 times $13 million is staggering, and I will assume that there are many other states that spend much more.

Society is very proud of the treatment it gives Seniors and pats its own back for the enormous effort it puts into the task. While society in general is determined to help Seniors grow OLD in relative physical comfort, it pays little or no attention to the mental needs of Seniors. Until the welfare state arrived, all such coddling was strictly voluntary. No one even dreamed of actually helping people age, but the welfare bureaucracy is replete with "experts" who are now making a career of teaching Seniors to lie down, roll over, and become dependent on them so they can have a job.

Society, for the most part, means well in all its efforts. Unfortunately, everything it does has an effect exactly opposite of what is apparently intended. Society tells us that we will be over the hill at 60 facing a dreary old age and that they are here to rescue us — until the undertaker rescues us from them evidently. Almost everything society would have us believe about our lives after 74 is untrue — except that we do die. I, for one, am not in favor of letting anyone tell me when I'm supposed to do that.

Like almost everyone else, I listened to this negative training. Scientists told us that by the time we reached 60, three-fourths of all our thinking had become negative. I knew I wasn't as happy as I had been at three, but everyone else was in the same fix. So I believed as they wanted me to, that it was an inevitable part of growing old and nothing could be done about it. Everyone had to grow old, and even though I didn't want to, I accepted that it must be.

I am proud to be in the 69% who have survived past 75, but I wandered around in this area for more than 10 years before I realized it was not just a temporary, overnight campground for wandering Gypsies, that it was the land the Creator had set aside for us surviving positive thinkers. I wanted to learn more.

When I began to think, really think, it became apparent to me that the colossal effort of society's well-meaning programs and myths was negative and depressing. I realized that what they say must happen to us all is what they call "the aging process," and it left virtually no room for the enormous exuberance and positiveness of the human spirit. Society's efforts on my "aging" behalf suddenly took on the specter of assisted, slow suicide.

"Grandpa's" Retirement

It was in New York in the mid-twenties. The retiree was a department head of a big insurance company. He was an "old" man of 60. Two or three of the near-top brass were MC's, and about 25 of the people he knew and a few wannabees, like the author, were there to hear him honored for his faithful service and to tell him that he was being rewarded for it by being allowed to now drop his burden which had grown too tough for him to handle at his advanced age. He was told that he was being turned out to pasture because that was more fitting for him than being sent to a glue factory.

The poor old fellow had been looking forward to that night for years. Now he could sit in the old rocking chair and rest and enjoy life until the end. That was all he and everyone there expected to happen. Everyone thought of it as the end for him, including himself. I thought of it as far worse than any funeral I had ever attended.

It was like all retirement banquets of that time. Often, the retirees died at the usual two weeks after a birthday or other big event.

Oh, yes. He was given the usual gold watch with his name engraved inside. Gold watches were always engraved. No one knew why they were engraved, other than it was considered proper, but heirs always had trouble selling them. Even in the 1920's, society was assisting slow suicides of its Senior Citizens.

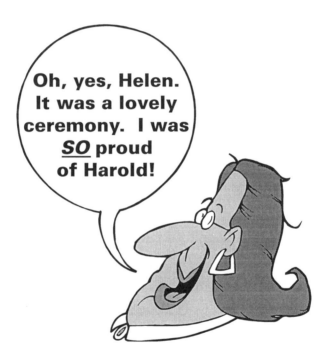

Grow Old — Stay Young
Your Choice

Instead of buying into what I discovered to be lies, I got busy, and I've done more thinking since I turned 90 than I did in the 90 years before. I started writing this book about staying young. I had had a belly full about how to grow old gracefully and graciously and in physical comfort with never a word about staying young and having fun. Not one book had ever been written on it that I could find. The Library of Congress has 94 books and 45,000 papers on GROWING OLD but not one on STAYING YOUNG!

Since there was apparently no other source, I dug over 250 ideas about staying young out of my head. I started exploring answers to questions like why we die at the average age of 74 and why women live longer than men. I knew there had to be answers, and I found them and dozens more. Every new idea was looked at from every angle and beaten to death and replaced by a better one. New ideas are born by doing that, and when you spend 1,000 hours a year looking for answers, you get pretty good at it. **Problems that look impossible to solve can usually be solved if you think long and hard and straight.**

For example, women used to have the same life expectancy as men, but now they are outliving men. The reason is simple: They expect to outlive men, so they do. Little girls are growing up being told they will live longer than men, and when they believe it, it becomes so. Another reason women outlive men is that, when a man retires and starts to rest and enjoy retirement, women go right on working and serving. They tend to their homes and families as they have always done and seldom make it to the rocking chair to while away the days with their husbands. They maintain their lifetime relationships and, if they have been working outside their homes for years, usually renew their interest in their homes. Retirement doesn't mean quitting to most women, and they seldom just sit and tear pages off the calendar waiting for "their time to go." Women, far more often than men, stay younger and live longer because they remain active and involved in the world around them, living life to its fullest.

> *At first, exploring your brain will be like going into an unlighted, mammoth cave with a book of matches to look for you don't know what.*

The first fact you find means nothing, but after you have found more, you begin to realize that all of them shed a little light on each other. Each new revelation is almost like a piece of a jigsaw puzzle, and soon you will be able to lay them out in some sort of picture. That helps in finding more pieces to fill the gaps. Each one lights up the others.

Quit worrying about what to do after 75, 85, or 100. You are entering a vast new world filled with hundreds of interesting problems that need to be solved. As you move forward, you will be able to see them more clearly and solve them more quickly and have the most thrilling fun you've ever had.

I have had more real fun in the 26 years since I passed 70 than in my first 70 years.

I'm expecting to live more and do more and have more fun in the next 24 than in the first 96. I may not make it all the way, but I'm sure having fun trying. My 80's and 90's have been more fun than my 60's when I was afraid to buy a green banana and take it home to ripen. I have no more worries.

I Think I Can!
I Think I Can!
I Think I Can!
I Think I Can!
I ~~Think~~ I Can!
Know

You learned the single greatest lesson in how to live a long, full life while you were a little child. Remember the little steam locomotive you used to imitate? It started out pulling a load by slowly saying, "I . . . think . . .I . . . can; I . . . think I . . .can; I think I . . . can"; and gradually it was going faster and faster, just like the steam locomotive of that day. Even if you never heard this lovely children's story, you can imitate the courageous little positive thinker by starting slowly saying, "I think I can; I think I can," and gradually picking up speed. Even the modern kid you are today can enjoy and learn from this most basic of premises — if you think you can, you can.

Very, very few of the things that make our lives more pleasant were discovered accidentally, such as rubber and penicillin. Nearly all were discovered by people saying, "I think I can; I think I can," and then setting out to prove it because they thought they could.

The awesome power of mental attitude was first revealed to me when my mother refused to die until she could say good-bye to all six of us kids. She was 76 and lived alone. Two strokes had paralyzed one side of her body and put her to bed permanently. She hated being dependent. She told my brother to call the siblings and tell them to come.

I was the last to arrive. Her doctor was just leaving, but he took me aside and told me that if I had not come for a year, she would have been waiting. He predicted that after she visited with me, she would be gone in two days.

My mother told me not to grieve for her, she had lived her life and was well pleased with it, but was tired and now was useless, so she was going to rest. She left us the next day with a smile on her face.

Nearly everyone knows of similar cases. But do you know that very few die just before a birthday? A great many, however, die just about two weeks after their birthday. That is by far the most popular and fashionable time to die, but one thing is certain: If you do not expect to live 100 years or 120 years, you will not, and it's an indisputable fact that if you die at 74, you are not going to have any fun at 96, as I am now having. That is why I expect to live more and accomplish more in the next 24 years than in the past 96. If I am still going strong at 120, I have an option to go for 970. The first person who breaks Methuselah's record of 969 years will be the first one who thinks he can.

Positive Future
Bright Future

It is almost impossible to be raised in this society and not believe that when you retire you're over the hill. That is evident when you see how many Seniors have bought prearranged funerals, complete with headstones with their names already inscribed, and are proud of it. They are entitled to be proud, provided they can forget that they did it and live their lives to the fullest, instead of waiting to occupy that burial plot and have the last date chiseled into the marble headstone. Those who cannot rid their minds of the fact that their funeral is all paid for seem to be destined to expedite their sad day of occupancy.

Like my friends, most of your friends who have died did so just about as they expected. Those of us who have reached 75, 85, 95, and so on, got here by always looking for the bright side of everything. There really is a bright side to everything: even death, so we have no fear of it. We know that the troubles we have ignored for years (thereby robbing them of most of the pain they would have given us otherwise) are gone forever. We are going to a better home, and we die only once. Why should we worry? The fun we are choosing to have, however, can continue because we are using the brains with which God has blessed us.

The most pitiable deaths among those who are in the 31% who reached 60 in good health and survived past 74 is the death of those whose brains die before their bodies do. That is perhaps the saddest part of the silly aging process, and it is mostly unnecessary, except for those suffering from Alzheimer's disease or maybe brain tumors. Brains for the most part do not wear out — they rust out from lack of use.

All of us positive thinkers know that our bodies can slow down but brains improve with use.

It is no wonder that so many brains rust out in light of the vast army of bureaucrats whose perks and pensions are dependent on our not using our own brains and relying on our own resources to remain independent. Except for cancer, accidents, and a few other things over which we have no control, people can live as long as they want to live provided they do something that gives them a reason to want to.

If you have quit thinking of 74 as OLD and started using the brain your Creator gave you, let's take a look at what the future may be expected to bring. I am awed and inspired by the fact that I have seen in my lifetime more than 45% of our country's history and well over half the technical progress made in the world since time began. I believe we are just on the brink of seeing unthinkable changes very soon that will make the changes that have come before seem almost insignificant. I wouldn't miss this "awakening" for the world.

The prospects for the future are so marvelous, I've decided to stick around to see it all unfold — and I intend to keep as many of you along for the ride as I can. About 1985, new phrases began creeping into the language. Neuro Linguistic Programming, Virtual Reality, and Fuzzy Logic are new worlds waiting to be explored and used. The fabulous world of goodies being discovered is, for the most part, right between our ears and will make the mountain of technical advances already found almost insignificant compared to what is coming. If you are not thrilled with all the prospective goodies about to come our way, call the undertaker and make room for fun-loving people.

Here we are on the entrance ramps to the fantastic information highway. It will be the biggest show the world has ever seen, and we have ringside seats, unencumbered by the necessity to make a living or raise children or rise to the top of the corporate ladder. I am looking forward to it. Why not make it even more memorable by recycling our brains and starting a new life exploring the 120 years our bodies are designed to last? And isn't it ironic that retirees who cannot find anything to do are dying of boredom?

In recent years, we have been so prosperous we have all gotten lazy, soft, and selfish and raised "me first" kids, many of whom never have learned how to work. These kids have been "trained" to believe that they are entitled to this, that, and everything they want. We are more divided now on everything than ever before. Some of it is spontaneous and self-ignited, but there is so much controversy over the size of everybody's slice of the pie that we have somehow forgotten to bake the pie. This war between the classes will be settled by nature's survival of the fittest. An empty belly is always an incentive to work.

Capital and labor are beginning to see that they both are in the same boat and are beginning to work together. That will continue and keep us alive in global competition.

I believe that the bitter fights now going on will fade away and we will come together as Americans. We will tackle the deficit by not borrowing money to waste and throw away. At the last minute of the last hour, we will keep our country from going down the drain. We will quit trying to carry water in a sieve. The money we waste, if used wisely, could pay our debt. Eventually we will learn and survive. We will do it by starting to vote again and bringing our government home from Washington and keeping it where we can watch it. We are not yet quite angry enough to get off our fannies and begin to govern our own future, but when we finally get tired of seeing arrogant bureaucrats steal our money, we will unleash all the pent up experience and knowledge, and we will stop it.

When We Do Go, What?

This book has shown you how to add half a century to your life. Now I will show you how to increase the odds of getting into Heaven while increasing your own self pride. No matter how much you have accomplished to be proud of, you can leave nothing more valuable after your death than an eye and organ donor card.

Every donor card is a potential ticket to the ultimate resting place. It just might be the thing that opens the Pearly Gates.

Many states now have laws that require hospitals, doctors, nurses, etc., who are losing a patient to request permission to "carve up" the deceased to supply parts to transplant into total strangers. Over the years, thousands of people have been requested to do that, and thousands have refused. The gruesome picture of having your loved one "carved up" is what the general public thinks of when they lose a loved one. It is so insensitive and the timing is so wrong that it must be the worst possible sales talk.

Another dream-big, reach-for-the-stars project that needs doing: Under the guise of protecting their privacy, a custom has arisen of keeping the names of organ donors and recipients secret from each other. Of course, in a few cases, everyone would agree it is necessary. It has, however, given the public the impression that it must somehow be wrong or it would not be kept in the closet. Add to that the gruesome reports of "organ selling," choosing one person to die before another so their organs can be used for some famous person, etc., that have built up over the years, and that adds up to the reality that only one donor is found in over half a million people. The truth of the matter is that both parties and both families involved in an organ transplant are benefitted and made proud, so hiding it makes it look bad and helps cut donors to 4500 a year.

If you want a powerful reason to go for 120, start looking for ways to end this silly practice by getting people to do their own thinking and realize the beauty of donating. A signed and witnessed donor card is a legal contract that should be carried out even if relatives object. The mere fact that medical personnel lean over backwards to be sure even one relative is not offended encourages objections. I hate to say it, but it also saves them work. They allow a relative to overrule the wishes of the deceased and ignore the plight of the possible recipients.

There are so many beautiful, positive, cheerful things about organ transplantation that it is a shame the same negative, gloomy attitude that surrounds aging has been built around it. Who wants to demolish that myth and show the happy, beautiful side that reaching for the stars will keep you young until the day you die smiling, before you get old, whether it be at 100, 120, or 970.

The time to get donors is while people are alive and well. You can sign an Eye (only the corneas are taken) and Organ Donor Card, get two witnesses, and it becomes a legal contract. However, I am told that many hospitals will not honor the expressed wish of the deceased if the relatives protest. That is hard to believe because it is so stupid. The fears of the relatives, spawned by years of stupid salesmanship, overlooks the wishes of the donor and the prayers of people whose lives can be saved by the donated organs. Is this just plain stupidity? Is there an ulterior motive? There could be. Anyway, it is time for us to find out. There are oodles of technical problems in all transplanting that limit the number that can be performed, so we must not let self-inflicted excuses interfere with the greatest gifts we can give. I do not believe that any donors are ashamed of their role nor the recipients of theirs.

In April 1992, Dear Abby published a beautiful letter from a mother who had lost a 19-year-old son in an auto accident and donated his kidneys to two people. One was a lady about 40, the other a 15-year-old boy. The mother and the two recipients searched for and found each other. The recipients were naturally profuse with their thanks for their lives, and the mother's pain was greatly eased. She was proud that parts of her son were still living and had saved two lives. Some people are very touchy about their privacy, but not nearly as touchy as the medical community would have us believe. Let's end this hush, hush about donating by encouraging people involved on both sides to get in touch with each other. Probably, nearly all will go for it and be much happier. The picture the public has of donating will be the positive, bright one, not the gruesome one they think of now.

It is my opinion that even cemeteries will soon come to an end. They serve no useful purpose and are costly in money and labor. We kid ourselves about "perpetual care." Why should I feel entitled to six feet of the world's surface forever? What have I done to entitle me to have someone mow the grass on my grave forever? What good does it do? Is the world better off because the grass is mowed on my grave? I doubt it. If you have done anything worth being remembered for, you will be remembered with or without a grave and monument. Tombstones never gave anyone immortality. To me, they are a waste, and funerals are a barbaric custom no longer serving a purpose — if they ever did. No matter what else you leave, the most important things are those parts of your body that are transplantable.

All of us are touched and a little envious when we read of some wealthy person's passing on and leaving a fortune to benefit other people not so well off. Danny Thomas told us, "It is not what you accumulate for yourself that matters, it is what you do for others." Most of us think, "How nice to be able to do that." Well, every one of us can leave something more precious than a fortune.

Don't ever get the idea that there is nothing you can do to help others. Each one of us is richer than we think. There are 25 parts of the human body that are now transplantable. No matter how old you are, your two corneas, tiny bits of tissue no bigger than a nail clipping from your little finger and no more important on the front of your eyeballs, can give sight to two blind people who never have seen their loved ones. The corneas are the only parts of the eyes touched, and their removal does not mar your appearance. Your skin can keep a badly burned baby or adult from horrible agony while they grow new skin. Your two kidneys can rescue two of the 30,000 people who are being kept alive by dialysis machines while praying for a new kidney. Your two lungs can restore two people to good health and a happy life. Your heart and liver and pancreas can keep their recipients alive and thanks God for your kindness. All of these, as well as your skin, bones, and other useable parts can long outlive you on this earth. As medical science advances, more and more organs will become transplantable. What could make you more proud and happy than helping relieve the pain and suffering of another human being or even extend the life of someone who will also die without your help? It seems to me that donating whatever of my body can be used by others is a lot better than burying them in a velvet- or satin-lined coffin.

Accentuate the Positive

Scientists have told us for a long time now that only 5% of the human brain has ever been used. For those who can recognize an opportunity when they see it, the human brain is a huge smorgasbord of opportunities to explore. It can continue to exist on hope alone if necessary. Most of our "civilization" is the product of an idea that originated in one person's head and was put to work.

Protecting the environment, curing polio, transplanting organs, persuading people to switch from negative to positive thinking and staying young instead of growing old, all started in one person's head, often a very ordinary, unspectacular individual. For instance, Helen Keller started the help for the blind. Rachel Carson's book *Silent Spring* started the movement to save our environment. The Wright Brothers' airplane brought us blessings that continue benefitting every person in the world. Martin Luther King, with one speech, changed the lives of every American. Lech Walesa started a labor movement that gets a huge share of the credit for overthrowing communism. Hopefully, this book will switch our country from negative thinking that considers GROWING OLD inevitable, to positive thinking about staying young and living as long as we can.

Henry Ford told us that some people think they can, others think they cannot. Both are right.

Breaking yourself of negative thinking can probably be done almost instantly by strong willed people. It will take time for others, largely because they do not consider it a bad habit and do not realize that it is keeping them from enjoying life to the fullest. These are the ones who are unwittingly choosing to die young instead of staying young.

The first thing necessary to become a positive thinker is to do a thorough housecleaning job on your brain.

You must rid it of a lifetime accumulation of negative, gloomy, and hopeless lies that society calls aging. All the negative thoughts have to be removed from your head and the place scrubbed and fumigated, or before long you will be back in the old rut that will lead directly to your grave. Get it completely out of your life and keep it out, or the enormous mass of it will overcome your efforts to acquire the habit of thinking positively. If you feel yourself slipping back into the old, negative rut, remember that that is the route taken by the 31% who deprive this earth and their families and friends of their presence too soon. Really, it does not take much will power to choose between staying young and dying young.

Now that the dismal mental swamp is cleared away, you are ready to start living as life is meant to be. Here's how!

If you have not already done so, the first step in breaking the bad habit of negative thinking is to pick a goal and go for it. It doesn't matter whether you go to 80, 100, 120, or 970. The cost is the same for all. When your goal is settled upon, the road ahead brightens immediately, and you can plan your life better. Also, a goal gives you an interest in life, without which no one lives long. Immediately, you quit wondering how long you are going to live and start making plans to do all those things you dreamed of doing but did not have time. You will begin to realize that you are never old until you think you are, that the best is yet to come. You learn that those who continue learning and thinking and sharing themselves with others continue living.

The first thing you will learn is that your bad habit of looking on the dark side is a lot worse than you ever realized, and you will wish that you had never started it. Don't waste any of your new positive-thinking time, however, fretting about it. Instead, try to avoid the words "old," "older," "aging," and similar words. Let them rest; they're worn out. Substitute words and thoughts of youth, growth, spring, joy, vigor, sunshine, and happiness.

Quit asking questions about people's health. Never give them a chance to reply, "As well as could be expected at my age," and decide not to answer questions about your own health with that sort of reply. Beat them to the punch by telling them how healthy they look. No matter if they do feel terrible, they will feel less terrible. You will have postponed their funeral a few minutes with one little ray of sunshine. You will have lightened their heavy burdens. Your sympathy would have added to their burdens.

Positive thinkers see a traffic light as a go light. Negative thinkers just see a stop light. Negative thinkers dread a dreary old age, part of their looking for the dark side of everything. They expedite their own funerals and all with whom they come in contact.

Consider the following examples:

POSITIVE ATTITUDE	NEGATIVE ATTITUDE
Optimistic	Pessimistic
Go light	Stop light
Glass half full	Glass half empty
Life begins at 65	Over the hill at 65
Better prepared to live now	Not much left in life but the old rocking chair
Sees retirement as a glorious opportunity to do all he's wanted to	Prearranges funeral — then starts looking forward to it
Exercises mind and muscle	Begins asking friends, "How are you feeling today?" They answer, "As well as can be expected." He tells them,

	"Better slow down. You're not so young anymore."
Stays busy, feels needed.	Worries about loss of memory, hearing, teeth, poor vision, impotence, pain, feebleness, arthritis, emphysema, etc.
Harnesses nature's strongest force, the will to survive	Sees only gloom and the grave and waits for the undertaker.
Quits using words like old and aging.	Speaks and thinks in terms of old and aging.
Starts exploring the fantastic smorgasbord of opportunities you helped create for everyone to enjoy.	R.I.P.
Tells friends he meets, "Gee, you are looking great. Isn't this a glorious day to enjoy life?"	
Sets a goal of 100 years or more and goes for it. Makes it and, boy, does he celebrate. What next? Methuselah's record of 969 years!	
Postpone your funeral	Expedite it

There are hundreds of overworked phrases that expedite but only a few that postpone funerals. "Have a good day" is the first you might think of. The negative thinkers in society are trying to abolish it by poking fun at it and calling it much overused. Actually, it should be used more often. We can add firepower to it by saying it this way: "Make yourself a great day!" It has more lift and would brighten your day and help keep everyone young. It will appeal to all — except maybe those among us who don't believe they are in control of creating good things for themselves.

Jack Benny had the right idea. He stayed 39 for years and years and years, then died young.

Avoid people who want to compare their ailments with yours. Their miseries are mostly between their ears. You can let them enjoy them without your help. These people's aches and pains are very contagious, and they make the communities where they live a warehouse for the soon dead. So steer clear and don't let yourself be sucked back in the negative thinking abyss. Most of the ailments that plague Seniors can be cured quickly by their getting off their fannies and going to work at anything useful that will give them an interest in life.

Avoid old people — even if they are only 40.

They are the ones who sit on their fannies wondering how long they are going to live and how dreary the old age that they expect is going to be. Their only hope is that the undertaker will come before life becomes unbearable. Stay as far away from these people as you can, whether they're 40 or 69. It is difficult — though not impossible — to maintain a positive mental attitude when in the company of such heavy negativity.

Don't expect to change the lifelong habit of looking for the dark side overnight. You will have to really work at it, but in due time, you will begin to realize that it is easier and more fun to be happy than miserable. Actually, the primary difference between positive and negative thinkers is the same as the difference between happiness and misery, between living and dying.

Staying young is a mental state of positive thinkers. Growing old is a physical state of negative thinkers.

If you are ever tempted to quit working toward a more positive attitude, remember that the 69% who choose life have a lot more fun than the 31% who choose the grave. So, if you can't cut the mustard by yourself, join a club and help one another do it faster and easier.

There are two ways to switch from negative thinking to positive, individually or with a club or group of people working towards the same goal. A reasonable amount of will power is needed if you do it as an individual. It is much quicker and easier (and more fun) if you do it as a group and help one another.

Neither way will succeed unless you first empty your mind of all the negative trash stored there. Clean, wash, and fumigate until the last lingering odor of negativity is gone before you start. Otherwise, the new knowledge you store there will be contaminated, and you will be back in the old rut again. The rut will become your grave.

The members of any club, like Kiwanis, can quit looking at the dark side and switch to looking at the bright, positive side of life. They can teach one another to become optimists instead of pessimists and end their present silly, stupid, senseless, nonproductive expediting of each other's funerals in six months, but only if they sincerely work at it.

Many clubs make a fun game out of fining members for certain offenses, like not wearing a badge or other more or less trumped up charges. It works fine as long as you keep it a fun game and members work overtime to devise clever ways to lay traps for one another to get them fined and provide a laugh for all. It can have a kick back if it puts emphasis on the fining rather than on the fun of devising clever schemes of entrapment. An overdose of fining tends to make some think they were being forced to do something. So keep it fun by elaborate entrapment schemes.

The idea of fining club members can help change the groups' negative energy to positive. Clubs can start by fining members for the use of a few words like OLD, OLDER, AGING, and that negative question, "How are you?" or the even worse reply, "As well as can be expected." Gradually, more and more negative ideas and phrases can be added to the prohibited list. Once members start looking for them, everyone will be amazed at the vast number of negative thoughts and ideas that all of us use to deprive ourselves and those around us of that half century of additional life that we are able to claim.

Whatever club will be the first to try it, sincerely try it, will succeed in enriching the everyday lives of all its members. The ripple effect of a movement like this will no doubt cause that club to be recognized as the leader, the first of a thousand, thousand points of light that changed this nation from looking with dread at dying soon after retirement to one of greeting retirement as the beginning of the harvest time of life that can last half a century or more.

Certainly, the first club that rids its members of negative thinking and has them looking forward to something wonderful will be remembered a long, long time. It is my opinion that this club will also attract more members from the positive thinking ranks than they know what to do with. As soon as other clubs and groups start seeing their members leaving for a more positive atmosphere, you can bet they will take a good look at changing their ways of thinking to entice their members back and gain new members themselves. All of them will be amazed to find out how positive action breeds positive thinking and how much everyone's life is improved by pulling their feet out of the negative muck and placing them on solid, positive ground. Negative thinking is just a bad habit indulged in by people too lazy to think or to observe the misery it causes themselves and those around them.

The job is open for anyone who wants it. The hours will be long. There will be no financial reward, but you will have an interest in life that is so great it will keep you alive until you are at least 120. Who knows, it might be great enough to last 970 years.

Take this idea to your own clubs and organizations. You may well be the catalyst for change that has been needed to get your friends out of the rut of looking back, remaining stagnant, or simply thinking there isn't much of a future after retirement. Can you imagine how good you would feel about yourself if you could do that for your club or organization and watch the fingers of light spreading throughout your community? You can do this and more — if you think you can. Ask Roger Bannister.

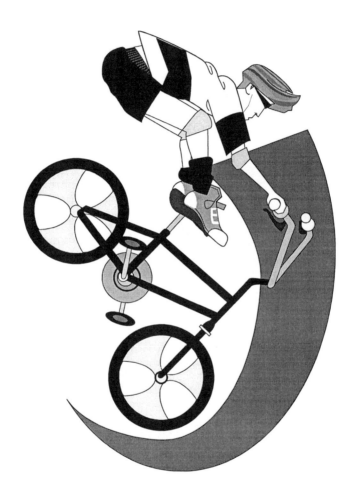

Just Look at the Kids!

If we start using a second 5% of our brain, we would probably double our degree of civilization and make ourselves more reluctant to leave our fantastic world. Many people are worried about the $5 trillion hole we have insisted on getting into. They need not be. Our present ability to think can pull us out if we use it. It will not strain our brains. Ordinary common sense can get us out of it. Millions of housewives have the know-how. All we need to do is use it. We will when we must.

One of the most amazing thing to me about our unused brain power is that 10-year-old kids are discovering physical and mental abilities we never knew we had. Watching them do things on skateboards, bicycles, surfboards, rollerblades, and all the other hitherto considered impossible fetes of the human body is thrilling. The gyrations these kids are achieving with their bodies and sports equipment would have been thought insane 20 years ago. The awesome power of mental attitude and believing you can is most apparent in the kids who are performing high-tech computer programming, breaking records almost as soon as they are made.

Our brains are computers and can be programmed by the "software" we choose to put into them. Software tells a computer what to do and it does it. You can program your brain to look on the positive side, the bright side, and it will do what it is told to do. You will be happier joining the 69% who survive long past 75 and enjoy their lives. You can also, however, program your brain to look for the negative, gloomy side, expedite your own demise, and join the 31% who make that choice. Think about it. Youngsters (no matter what age) look forward. Oldsters (no matter what age) look back too much, and their looking forward is confined to the good rest they intend to have for a few years before going to their inevitable grave. They spend too much time GROWING OLD and not enough in living. That is, unfortunately, their decision.

Okay, Positive Ain't Perfect

I know what you're thinking, and you're right. The world is full of irritants for Seniors, and the worst of all are the little ones. They are usually so trivial that you pay no conscious attention to them as they annoy you, because if they were bigger, you would do something to end them. Here are a few examples of my own irritants:

Buttoning tiny buttons with arthritic fingers
Undershirts, etc., that are put on over the head
Bending far enough to tie shoelaces
Trimming toe nails
Eyes that are slower to adjust to light changes
Hearing aids that plug up with wax
Hearing aids that amplify unwelcome noises and
    drown out conversations

I'm sure you can add to this list more irritants that annoy you. As the years pass by, more and more such petty and trivial irritants appear. They can be ignored and over-looked and life enjoyed in spite of them, or they can be magnified and make you miserable. **The choice is yours.** When your own mental attitude is in command, you can choose to quit paying attention to them, and, almost mi-raculously, most of them will disappear.

Positive thinkers will focus on the joys of false teeth compared to natural teeth that the dentist insisted on sav-ing, thereby risking abscesses that could kill and are often the cause of arthritis. Of course, dentists would be horri-fied if too many knew this. They, too, must eat. But one man's experience, mine, will not put them out of business.

If you travel a lot, you will encounter lots of things that can ruin your fun — if you let them. You can dodge some of them yourself, and others you can make the hotel remedy. For instance, most hotels are air conditioned. All that means is that they keep running the same air through the air conditioners and never admit any fresh air. It cuts their electric bill. If they have one central system, there is no way you can tell, except you may not be able to sleep. If each room has its own air conditioner or heat pump, most of them will have a fresh air vent that can be opened or closed, and maids always close them. Many hotels take the knobs off the controls to prevent the vents being opened. Usually, needle-nosed pliers will open them. There is a sure way to find out if the vent is closed. Hold a piece of Kleenex by one corner and move it all over the surface of the outside of the unit. If the vent is open and the unit operating, the Kleenex will be sucked against the unit. That works only on the ground floor, usually. Better yet, tell the management to open the vent or hunt another motel. If there isn't one, pull the unit out of the wall and open the vent.

Often, the reading light is 40 watt. Carry your own with you. Start with two because you will forget in the beginning and leave the first one. A reading light that enables you to read in bed and that can be turned on and off without getting out of bed is nice, and the price you pay has little to do with what you get. Light switches one-quarter inch in diameter that have to be twisted are a sure indication that the motel owner does not have arthritis in his fingers. There are lots of other little annoyances in motels that could ruin your stay if you let them, so ignore them.

Another irritant is auto mechanics who do not realize that we have owned several cars during our lives and worn out most of them. My experience has been that they think I'm too old to know that I don't need an engine overhaul when one spark plug has gone bad. I tell them that is exactly what I thought was wrong, thank them, and tell them I will be back next week and let them overhaul that engine. The more irritants you can turn into fun, the happier you will be and the longer will live.

The principal irritant that all Seniors face is the large segment of the population that simply assumes everyone has to grow old and life is all downhill after 60, that your brain died the day you retired, and that it is inevitable and happens to everyone. Don't let it get your goat. I run into this unthinking attitude toward older people constantly. A small percentage think I should get out of their way by dying and are actually hostile toward me. They assume that my brain is dead, and I know theirs was never more than 10% alive. So pity them and the undertaker who has to decide whether or not they are alive or dead when he is called to bury them.

When you encounter this sort of ignorance and if

you haven't had your allotment of fun that day, there is no harm in verbally removing a chunk of the well-meaning though misinformed person's hide. Rather than let his rude and insensitive behavior bother you, you can turn it into great entertainment for yourself. Don't be surprised, though, if he seems unable to grasp that he has been had by a Senior citizen.

Frequently, I go to meetings of retirees and sit down at a table for eight and introduce myself to those on either side of me. Many times, I am left out of the discussions and no one asks my opinion. Think about it. I'm 96; most of them are young retirees of 65 to 70. Without even talking to me, they write me off because of their perception that I couldn't possibly have anything to offer to the conversation. It gives me a good chance to see whether they know what is going on in the world. They do not make me angry. They teach me more about human nature. They mean no harm. Occasionally, I get a chance to let them know I am still a living, breathing person. More often than not, if I see them again, they treat me normally. I let them dig their own graves if they insist. I will never let them dig mine.

We Haven't Seen Anything Yet!

Our world has changed more in my lifetime than in the 1000 years before, and it is just beginning to accelerate. We are seeing the blessings brought by fierce global competition, made possible by the airplane and rapid communication. The Japanese awakened us. Our business managers are beginning to realize that workers have brains and are learning how to get them to produce their best work by rewarding them.

Already more and more corporations are getting 25% to 50% of their profits from things that did not exist 5 or 10 years ago. All progress is brought about by competition. It, too, is speeding up, so hold onto your hats. Our world is changing faster and faster. Will we make as much progress in the next 169 years? Undoubtedly we will make more. Humans are not nearly as reluctant to think as they were before 1829. Thinking long, hard, and straight solves all problems. Your brain will not be overworked when you choose whether to die young or stay young and have fun.

For instance, try to find the reason why one person in every 3961 is over 100 in Iowa, while in Utah it is 1 in

19,338 and in Alaska it is 1 in 36,370. Everyone can figure out Alaska. Anyone over 74 who is not an Eskimo wouldn't go that far north. But Iowa and Utah will give your brains some healthy exercise, even if you do not solve it. Very few brains wear out; oodles of them rust out.

We Seniors are in an enviable position of being able to alter society's attitude about aging. There are sure signs of a positive change. Even though it is very subtle and not happening nearly fast enough, it is happening. Five years ago when I asked an audience, "How many of you are going for 100?" I got maybe one or two hands raised, and a whole lot of "Ha Ha's." I quit asking. But recently, I asked 50 or 60 Shriners that same question, and nearly every hand went up immediately.

Before the first airplane flew on December 17, 1903, barriers like national boundaries, oceans, and mountains had prevented workers in remote places from competing with other workers elsewhere in the world. Suddenly, airplanes were able to fly into those areas, and the Air Age was born. We learned that the tougher competition is, the better.

THE YOUNG METHUSELAH CLUB

CR

There is a giant sequoia in
California that is believed to be the
oldest living tree on earth.
Its name is Methuselah.

℘

At this writing, The Young Methuselah Club has one charter member, me. I believe it is time for all of us positive thinkers to get to know each other and gain strength and vitality
from the sharing of our positive selves with society. We need
to. We must be the catalyst that moves society out of the negative stance in which it is entrenched regarding its Seniors. It is
our duty, and perhaps our payment for the huge debt we will
leave, to make every effort to keep young people today from
being brainwashed with the same dreadful myths of aging that
have been perpetuated through the centuries. We are their hope,
and we number plenty to make an impact on the consciousness
of our society in general.

We must show the naysayers who would have us roll over
and be (not play) dead that associating with positive people is
more fun than associating with people who spend their lives
comparing aches and pains with their neighbors' miseries, and
that by doing so, we help each other stay young. Then and only
then can the time and effort and compassion that are now being
wasted helping all of us to be comfortable in our old age be
spent on the truly worthwhile endeavors of helping those who

can't help themselves and searching for even more of the wonders this world has available to us.

As more retirees are moving into retirement communities where everyone is near the same age, our youngsters are losing touch with society's elders, the very people from whom they must learn how to live their own lives.

The beliefs of The Young Methuselah Club are simple and straightforward (see next page).

The Club will have a newsletter filled with positive picker-uppers and only the sunny side of life. It will not be a bulletin board of ailments like arthritis, nor will the Club meetings be a place for "old people" to compare their aches and pains and miseries, especially those between their ears. For a few years yet, society will continue to manufacture gloom and assist people in "aging," but it is within our power to make that change happen much sooner than it will if we don't try.

Together we can build an organization that is dedicated to educating, improving, enhancing, and making more mentally healthy the day-to-day lives of all of our citizens, no matter what age. We can have an organization that will focus on the multitude of positive aspects of retirement, thereby enticing the 31% we are losing now to stick around and enjoy the roller coaster ride with us. We can make businesses, educators, medical personnel, and bureaucrats wake up their brains to interact with ours that have never slept to improve our society for us all.

I want to know who you are. I want to know all about you, your dreams, your goals, how you keep yourself positive, what contributions you are making, how you handle retirement irritants positively, and how you want to be involved in The Young Methuselah Club. After all, you are accepting the task of taking our positive message into your community. That makes you someone worth knowing.

So, come and join me in this Stay Young Land. With apologies to Robert Browning, I invite you to:

"Stay young along with me,
The best is yet to be,
The last of life for which the first was made."

BELIEFS OF THE YOUNG METHUSELAHS

The Young Methuselah Club is for people who
believe in better tomorrows because:

We have learned in life's boot camp how to get things
by first thinking how to do it, then doing it.

We agree with Shad Helmstetter that nothing is more
impossible than you think it is.

We know that there are two sides to everything. The
bright side brings happiness, the dark side misery.

We agree with Lincoln that most people are about as
happy as they make up their minds to be.

We like to be with other people like ourselves
who solve life's problems by thinking through
to the best solution.

We know some problems may have no known solution.
We know that ignoring or laughing at such problems
make them much less painful or annoying.

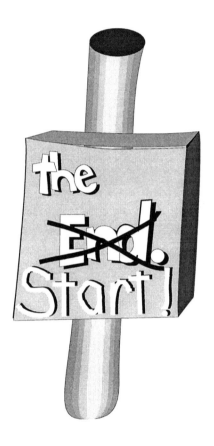

If you are a positive thinker like me and like to look ahead to a better future, I want you to join **The Young Methuselah Club** so we can plan and work together to build a better life for us all.

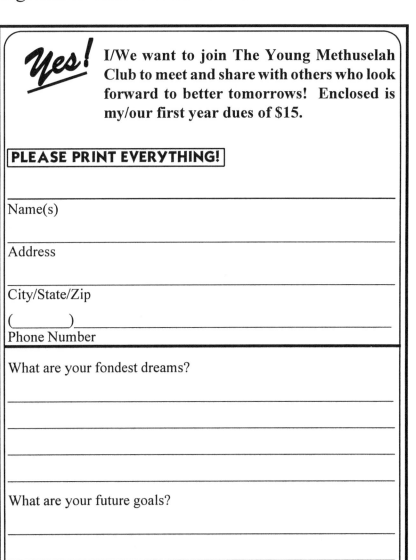

Yes! I/We want to join **The Young Methuselah Club** to meet and share with others who look forward to better tomorrows! **Enclosed is my/our first year dues of $15.**

PLEASE PRINT EVERYTHING!

Name(s)

Address

City/State/Zip

( )
Phone Number

What are your fondest dreams?

What are your future goals?

How do you keep yourself(ves) positive?

_____

_____

_____

How do you handle retirement irritants?

_____

_____

_____

How do you contribute to your community?

_____

_____

_____

What are your hobbies and/or interests?

_____

_____

How would you like to be involved in **The Young Methuselah Club**?

_____

_____

Complete and mail with $15* dues to:
Mr. E.L. Stephenson
3348 #38 North Thompson Street
Springdale, Arkansas 72764
(501) 750-1236

*We are hoping to never raise this fee!

ABOUT THE AUTHOR

E.L. "Steve" Stephenson was born December 16, 1899, in Carthage, Missouri, the fifth of six children. He grew up on farms in Fredonia, Kansas, and Antlers, Oklahoma. He attended the University of Kansas at Hays, Kansas, until he enlisted in the Marine Corps and went through boot camp at Parris Island, South Carolina.

Mr. Stephenson received his law degree from the University of Michigan Law School in 1922, but he never took the bar exam so that no one could call him a lawyer. From 1922 until 1970 when he "retired," he successfully worked for and managed several insurance company offices in Detroit, Lansing, Flint, Indianapolis, Louisville, and New York, as well as later building his own Aviation Insurance Agency in Chicago, insuring only airports and aircraft.

Steve flew for 41 years and owned four Cessnas from 1954 until 1970. He knows he has over 4000 hours of flight time and that none of it is "Parker Pen time." He literally made a living at his hobby and says, "That's the best way to go."

He pulled an Airstream trailer until 1977, when he bought a motor home that he still lives in today. According to him, it beats a tent or a penthouse in New York.

Steve joined the Toastmasters Club, #7304, and has made more than 100 speeches on "Staying Young, Staying Busy, and Staying Alive" to luncheon clubs in Northwest Arkansas.

Steve was married for 25 years to four different wives. Fourteen of those years were gloriously happy. Says he, "I cannot stand dumb women, and the smart ones think I need a boss." He has a dinner date scheduled with his editor on his 100th birthday, at which time they will surely establish a tradition that will be carried on for the next 20 and beyond.